External Fixation of the Pelvis and Extremities

External Fixation of the Pelvis and Extremities

Samir Mehta, MD
Department of Orthopaedic Surgery
University of Pennsylvania
Philadelphia, PA

Wudbhav N Sankar, MD
Department of Orthopaedic Surgery
University of Pennsylvania
Philadelphia, PA

Christopher T Born, MD, FAAOS, FACS
Professor of Orthopaedic Surgery
Temple University School of Medicine
Co-Director of Orthopaedic Trauma
Temple University Health System
Philadelphia, PA

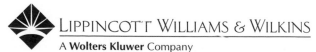

LIPPINCOTT WILLIAMS & WILKINS
A **Wolters Kluwer** Company
Philadelphia · Baltimore · New York · London
Buenos Aires · Hong Kong · Sydney · Tokyo

Managing Editor: Jennifer Jett
Cover Designer: Lou Moriconi
Compositor: Maryland Composition, Inc.
Printer: Walsworth

530 Walnut St.
Philadelphia, PA 19106 USA
www.LWW.com

Printed in the United States of America

Library of Congress Cataloging-in-Publication Data

Mehta, Samir.

External fixation of the pelvis and extremities / Samir Mehta, Wudbhav N. Sankar, Christopher T. Born.
   p. ; cm.
 Includes bibliographical references.
 ISBN 0-7817-6243-X
 1. External skeletal fixation (Surgery)--Handbooks, manuals, etc. I. Sankar, Wudbhav N. II. Born, Christopher. III. Title.
   [DNLM: 1. External Fixators--Handbooks. 2. Fracture Fixation--methods--Handbooks. 3. Dislocations--surgery--Handbooks. 4. Fractures--surgery--Handbooks. WE 39 M4985h 2005]
 RD103.E88M448 2005
 617.1'58--dc22
                                    2004021918

Care has been taken to confirm the accuracy of the information presented and to describe generally accepted practices. However, the authors, editors, and publisher are not responsible for errors or omissions or for any consequences from application of the information in this book and make no warranty, expressed or implied, with respect to the currency, completeness, or accuracy of the contents of the publication. Application of this information in a particular situation remains the professional responsibility of the practitioner.

The authors, editors, and publisher have exerted every effort to ensure that drug selection and dosage set forth in this text are in accordance with current recommendations and practice at the time of publication. However, in view of ongoing research, changes in government regulations, and the constant flow of information relating to drug therapy and drug reactions, the reader is urged to check the package insert for each drug for any change in indications and dosage and for added warnings and precautions. This is particularly important when the recommended agent is a new or infrequently employed drug.

Some drugs and medical devices presented in this publication have Food and Drug Administration (FDA) clearance or limited use in restricted research settings. It is the responsibility of the health care provider to ascertain the FDA status of each drug or device planned for use in their clinical practice.

The content expressed is the opinion of the authors and not necessarily that of Stryker Corp. This document is for educational use only. The information presented is intended to demonstrate a Stryker product. Always refer to the package insert, product label and/or instructions before using any Stryker product. Products may not be available in all markets. Product availability is subject to the regulatory or medical practices that govern individual markets. Please contact your Stryker representative if you have questions about the availability of Stryker products in your area.

Surgeons must always rely on their own clinical judgment when deciding which product and/or techniques to use with patients.

10 9 8 7 6 5 4 3 2 1

Table of Contents

Introduction
Basics of External Fixation   vii

Section 1: Upper Extremity   1

Chapter 1   Humeral Shaft Fractures   1

Chapter 2   Peri-articular Elbow Fractures and Dislocations   7

Chapter 3   Forearm Fractures   15

Chapter 4   Wrist Fractures   25

Chapter 5   Hand Fractures   33

Section 2: Pelvis   41

Chapter 6   Pelvic Fractures   41

Section 3: Lower Extremity   47

Chapter 7   Femoral Shaft Fractures   47

Chapter 8   Peri-articular Knee Fractures and Dislocations   53

Chapter 9   Tibial Shaft Fractures   61

Chapter 10   Peri-articular Ankle Fractures and Dislocations   69

Chapter 11   Forefoot Fractures and Dislocations   79

Glossary   87

References   88

Basics of External Fixation

External fixation refers to the technique of fracture fixation in which the orthopedic surgeon places pin clusters in separate fracture fragments and then connects the pin clusters to external bars to maintain the fracture in a desired spatial relationship.

Advantages

Despite the advent of new open reduction and internal fixation techniques including intramedullary devices, external fixation continues to have significant clinical appeal because of the following advantages:

(a) low-risk, stable fixation to traumatized surrounding soft tissues and bone
(b) straightforward and rapid application of device with minimal surgical blood loss
(c) minimally invasive technique preserving osseous blood supply
(d) adjustability with respect to translation, rotation, angulation, and axial alignment
(e) access to soft tissues for subsequent procedures and wound care
(f) ability for use as definitive fixation or as a temporizing device

(g) can be tailored to accommodate regional anatomy and a variety of pathologic lesions

Indications

The primary indications for external fixation include, but are not limited to:

(a) open fractures
(b) closed fractures with significant soft tissue injury
(c) periarticular fractures and joint dislocations
(d) unstable patients requiring rapid treatment of multiple injuries
(e) bone or soft tissue infection

Frame Design

External fixators in which pins are all inserted in the same plane are called uniplanar. When half-pins are inserted into two planes from one side of the limb, the fixation is biplanar. Ring fixators use frame components that pass around the limb and allow pins or transfixion wires to be inserted from multiple directions, allowing for treatment of significantly comminuted fractures and for multiplanar adjustments, but these fixators can obstruct soft tissue access. The hybrid external fixators combine some of the advantages of the uniplanar and multiplanar external fixator, allowing stabilization of periarticular fractures with less complexity than a ring fixator.

Frame Construction

To assemble an external fixator, stainless steel or titanium pins are first inserted percutaneously to obtain bicortical purchase within each of the fracture fragments. Pins are now available with hydroxyapitate coating allowing for improved bone ingrowth and better fixation. Specific insertion sites for the pins are based on not only the fracture pattern but also the regional neurovascular anatomy. The second basic component used in an external fixator is a clamp connecting the inserted pins to carbon fiber rods or rings. Finally, carbon fiber rods or rings are placed within the clamps, the fracture is reduced, and the construct is locked in place. Care is taken not to place the externals bars too close to the soft tissue to allow for wound care and swelling.

Biomechanics of Frame Constructs

External fixator frames should be assembled with some basic biomechanical principles in mind. The goal is to maximize the stiffness of the construct, thereby minimizing interfragmentary motion. Pin size, pin number, pin separation, pin proximity to the fracture, and bone-to-clamp distance all influence final mechanical stability.

Pin size

The bending and torsional strength of a pin varies by the radius of the pin to the fourth power. For example, a 6-mm pin (with a 3-mm radius) will have a bending and torsional stiffness five-times greater than a 4-mm pin (with a 2-mm radius). However, use of too large a pin will result in a stress riser and compromise the strength of the bone, leading to iatrogenic fractures. Transfixing pins, with centrally placed threads, are also available in varying sizes for improved construct stability.

Pin number

Increasing the number of pins in each major fragment reduces the stresses at each individual pin-bone interface. There are practical limits to the number of pins that can be placed within a fragment without compromising bone strength.

Pin separation and pin proximity to the fracture

The ideal position for pin placement is a near–far construct, with a pin placed close to the fracture site on both sides and a pin placed as far away as possible. Minimum distance between the pins closest to the fracture site is generally constrained by the quality and integrity of the bone adjacent to the fracture site and the minimum amount of bony margin that the orthopaedic surgeon deems necessary to prevent pin migration into the fracture site. Violation of this "zone of injury" or pin placement too close to the margins of the wound can lead to direct bacterial infection.

Bone-to-clamp distance

The distance from the surface of the bone to the connecting rod (i.e., bone-to-clamp distance) is inversely proportional to the stiffness of the construct.

Moving a clamp closer to the bone will increase the stiffness by a third-power relationship. Bone-to-clamp distance is constrained by the need to leave sufficient clearance for soft tissue swelling at the fracture site.

Management

The duration of external fixation is determined by the underlying role of the fixator. A temporizing external fixator can be used for a short period of time until soft tissues have stabilized sufficiently for definitive fixation. Conversion to an intramedullary device within the first 7 days of external fixation can be performed with lower risk of infection. External fixators can, of course, be used as definitive treatment, in which case the application may last longer depending on individual healing. Healing times can be decreased by reducing the frame stiffness during fracture consolidation through a process called dynamization. Dynamization of the external fixator is the conversion of a statically locked construct to one that allows load-sharing and micromotion.

Complications

Neurovascular injury can occur if the surgeon is not familiar with regional cross-sectional anatomy and the relative safe zones and danger zones for pin insertion. Overly rigid constructs can "unload" the fracture site, leading to weak endosteal callous formation and potential delayed or nonunions. If union does occur, the endosteal callous is at a higher risk for refracture because of the rigidity of the construct. Dynamization can speed union rate and improve the quality of bone formation.

The most common complication of external fixation, and potentially the most severe, is pin tract infection, which is thought to occur in between 0.5% and 10% of patients. It should be noted that all pin sites will have some drainage, and a spectrum of infection exists from minor inflammation remedied by local would care to osteomyelitis requiring irrigation and debridement. To minimize the risk of pin tract infections, all pins require "pin care," which consists of half-strength hydrogen peroxide and saline applied to the pin-soft tissue interface three times daily. If a large amount of drainage is occurring or if there is increased pain around the pin, then the patient should be started on an oral cephalosporin. Deeper infections, noted by purulent drainage, swelling, cellulites, and/or pin loosening, will require removal of infected pins, debridement, curettage, and open packing in addition to intravenous antibiotics. New pins may need to be placed at additional sites if the fracture has not healed.

Summary

As long as proper biomechanical principles are used and strict postoperative care issues are addressed, external fixation is an effective technique for the management of fractures and dislocations, especially when there is concern for soft tissues and minimally invasive surgery.

Frame configurations as shown are only suggested frame configurations. Pin placements as shown are for illustrative purposes only. Actual external fixation frame configurations and pin placements will be dependent on the clinical situation, local anatomy and the surgeon's discretion. If uncertainty exists with regard to the anatomical location of the neurovascular structures, the device should be used with extreme caution. Under these circumstances, the pins should be inserted under direct vision.

Chapter 1:
Humeral Shaft Fractures

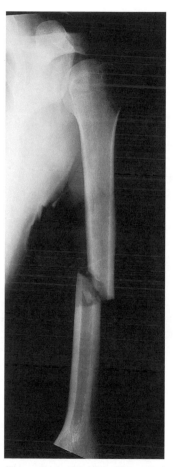
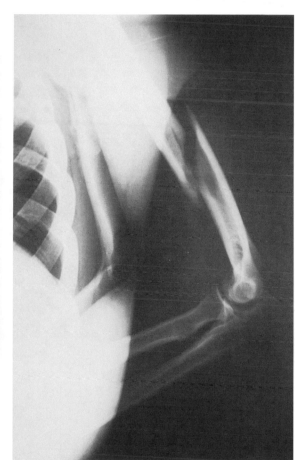

(From Craig FV, MD. *Clinical Orthopedics.* Baltimore: Williams & Wilkins, 1999.)

Epidemiology
- 3% of all fractures

Mechanism of injury
- Bending (e.g., MVA)
  - Most common
  - Transverse
  - Comminuted
- Torsion (e.g., fall on outstretched arm)
  - Usually in elderly
  - Spiral
  - Oblique

Clinical care
- Assess neurovascular status
  - Radial nerve
    - Holstein-Lewis
      Distal third humeral shaft fracture
      Classically associated radial nerve palsy
  - Median nerve
  - Ulnar nerve
  - Radial and Ulnar arteries
- Assess soft tissue injury
- Monitor compartments

Radiographic evaluation
- Full-length AP and lateral views of humerus
- Full shoulder and elbow radiographs
- Traction radiographs may aide in fracture definition
- CT/MRI rarely indicated unless pathologic fracture suspected

Nonoperative treatment
- Most often managed non-operatively
- Union rates 90%
- Hanging arm cast or coaptation splint for closed fractures meeting the following criteria
  - 3 cm of shortening
  - Less than 30-degree varus/valgus angulation
  - Less than 20-degree anterior/posterior angulation
- Conversion to functional brace within 1 to 2 weeks

HUMERAL SHAFT FRACTURES

Classification system

Descriptive classification system used most commonly

- Anatomic location
  - Proximal third
  - Middle third
  - Distal third
- Presence of comminution or butterfly
- Configuration
  - Transverse
  - Spiral
  - Oblique
  - Segmental
- Angulation
  - Varus/valgus
  - Anterior/posterior
- Translation (percentage of cortical contact)
- Shortening
- Open versus closed

Anatomy

- Shaft extends from the pectoralis major insertion to the supracondylar ridge
- Cross-sectional shape changes from cylindrical proximally to triangular distally
- Axillary nerve often 5 to 6 cm inferior to tip of the acromion
- Surrounded by two compartments
  - Anterior (e.g., median nerve, biceps, musculocutaneous nerve, brachial artery, ulnar nerve)
  - Posterior (e.g., triceps, radial nerve)
- Blood supply
  - Branches of brachial artery
    - Nutrient artery enters medially
- Radial nerve at risk as it courses within the spiral groove

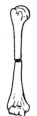

▲**Figure 2.** Nondisplaced transverse midshaft humerus fracture

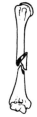

▲**Figure 3.** Translated spiral fracture with a butterfly fragment

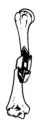

▲**Figure 4.** Severely comminuted midshaft humerus fracture

Figures 2–4: (From Craig EV, MD. *Clinical Orthopedics.* Baltimore: Williams & Wilkins, 1999.)

Model configuration

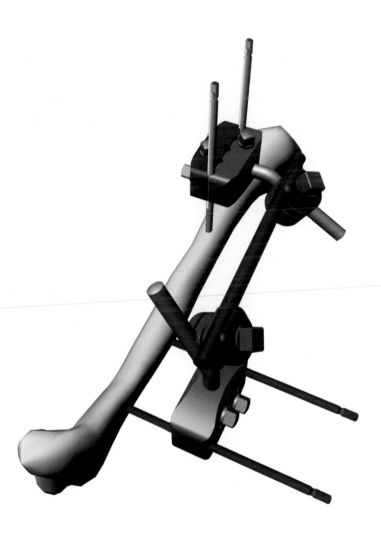

Pin placements as shown are for illustrative purposes only. Actual external fixation frame configurations and pin placements will be dependent on the clinical situation, local anatomy and the surgeon's discretion.

Safe zones and pitfalls

External fixation for the humerus is generally reserved in patients with severe soft tissue damage, multiply injured patients, open fractures with gross contamination, and infection.

- Proximal third (see "A" below)
  - Majority of neurovascular structures are located medially
    - Brachial artery and vein
    - Median and ulnar nerve
  - Half-pins are placed through anterolateral fibers of deltoid
    - Care is taken not to penetrate medial cortex
    - Axillary nerve at risk from proximal pins

- Middle third (see "B" below)
  - Half-pins placed anteriorly
    - Care is taken to not penetrate posterior cortex where radial nerve courses in spiral groove
- Distal third (see "C" below)
  - Half-pins or transfixation pins placed into lateral epicondyle (in a posterior oblique direction)
    - Avoid olecranon fossa and radial nerve
  - For transfixation pins, ulnar nerve at risk posterior to medial epicondyle
  - Place pins medial to lateral

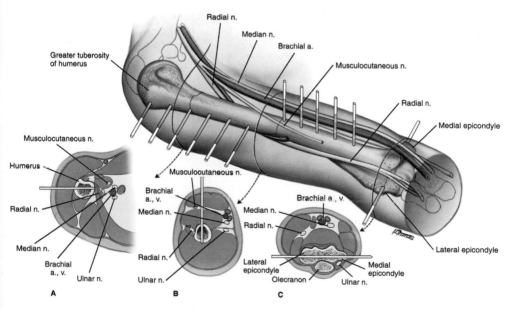

(From Hoppenfeld, S, MD; DeBoer, P, MA, FRCS. *Surgical Exposures in Orthopedics: The Anatomic Approach, 3rd Edition.* Philadelphia: Lippincott Williams & Wilkins, 2003.)

External fixator construct components

8-mm Connecting rod	1
4-mm half-pin	4
Multi-pin clamp assembly	2
30-degree Angled post	2
Rod-to-rod clamp	2

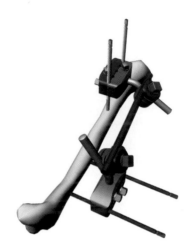

Alternative configurations

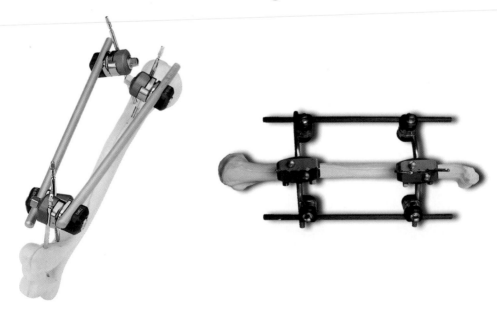

Pin placements as shown are for illustrative purposes only. Actual external fixation frame configurations and pin placements will be dependent on the clinical situation, local anatomy and the surgeon's discretion.

Chapter 2:
Peri-articular Elbow Fractures and Dislocations

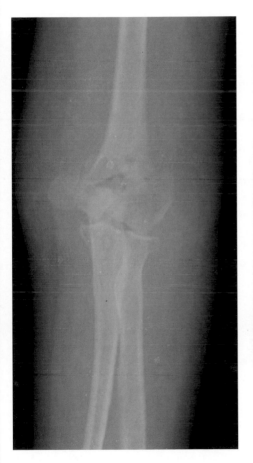
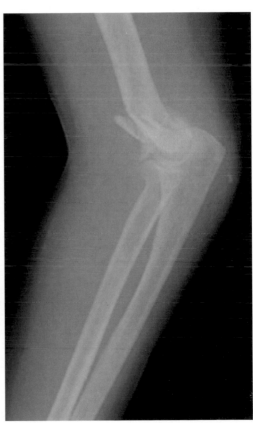

Epidemiology

- Supracondylar humerus fractures
  - Uncommon
  - 4.3% of all fractures
  - More than 80% are extension type
- Elbow dislocations
  - 11% to 28% of all injuries to elbow
  - Associated fractures
    - Radial head 5% to 11%
    - Medial or lateral epicondyle 12% to 34%
    - Coronoid process 5% to 10%
- Olecranon fractures
  - Bimodal distribution by age
- Complex elbow injuries may include dislocation with multiple associated fractures

Mechanism of injury

- Supracondylar humerus fractures
  - Extension (e.g., fall on outstretched hand)
  - Flexion
    - Axial load to elbow flexed more than 90 degrees
- Elbow dislocations
  - Usually result from fall on outstretched hand
  - Posterolateral dislocation results from
    - Elbow hyperextension
    - Valgus stress
    - Arm abduction
    - Forearm supination
  - Anterior dislocation
    - Direct force striking posterior forearm with elbow flexed
- Olecranon fractures
  - Direct
    - Fall on elbow flexed less than 90 degrees
    - Typically comminuted
  - Indirect
    - Fall on outstretched hand with sudden contraction of triceps
    - Usually results in transverse or oblique fractures

Clinical care

- Assess neurovascular status
  - Brachial artery
  - Median, radial, and ulnar nerves
- Closed reduction if necessary (reassess neurovascular status)
- Assess soft tissue injury
- Monitor compartments pressures

Radiographic evaluation

- Full-length AP and true lateral views of the elbow
- Traction x-rays often helpful in cases of intraarticular comminution
- X-rays after elbow reduction help identify associated fractures
- CT extremely useful to delineate intraarticular fracture pattern
- MRI can be used to evaluate elbow ligaments
- Arteriogram if arterial injury suspected

Nonoperative treatment

- Supracondylar humerus fractures rarely treated conservatively
  - Posterior long arm splint indicated for closed, nondisplaced fractures
  - Conversion to a long arm cast followed by early range of motion
- Elbow dislocations
  - Urgent closed reduction
  - Reassess neurovascular status
  - Range elbow to assess stability and presence of mechanical block such as intraarticular loose bodies
    - For stable elbows, a posterior splint at 90 degrees of flexion is used, followed by early range of motion
- Olecranon fractures
  - Long arm cast suitable for closed, nondisplaced fractures
  - Immobilize in 45 to 90 degrees of elbow flexion, followed by early motion

Classification systems

- Supracondylar humerus described by AO Müller classification (Figure 2)
  - Type A: Extraarticular
  - Type B: Unicondylar
  - Type C: Bicondylar
- Elbow dislocation
  - Descriptive classification system used most commonly (Figure 3)
    - Position of ulna relative to humerus
      Posterior (most common)
      Anterior
      Medial
      Lateral
      Divergent
  - Instability scale of Morrey
    - Type I: Posterolateral rotatory instability
    - Type II: Perched condyles with varus instability
    - Type IIIa: Posterior dislocation: valgus instability
    - Type IIIb: Posterior dislocation: grossly unstable
- Olecranon fractures—Schatzker (descriptive) classification (Figure 4)
  - Transverse (avulsion type occurring at sigmoid notch)
  - Transverse—impacted
  - Oblique—hyperextension
  - Comminuted
  - Oblique—distal
  - Fracture dislocation

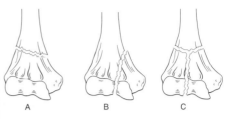

▲**Figure 2.** AO MüllerA types A, B, and C supracondylar humerus fractures (From Bucholtz RW, Heckman, JD, MD. *Rockwood & Green's Fractures in Adults, 5th Edition.* Philadelphia: Lippincott Williams & Wilkins, 2002.)

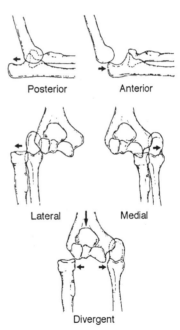

Posterior   Anterior

Lateral   Medial

Divergent

▲**Figure 3.** Elbow dislocations (From Koval KJ, MD, Zuckerman JD, MD. *Handbook of Fractures, 2nd Edition.* Philadelphia: Lippincott Williams & Wilkins, 2001.)

UPPER EXTREMITY

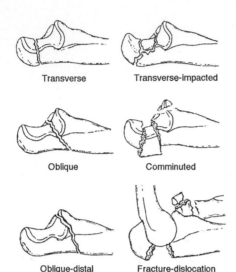

Transverse   Transverse-impacted

Oblique   Comminuted

Oblique-distal   Fracture-dislocation

▲**Figure 4.** Olecranon fractures (From Koval KJ, MD, Zuckerman JD, MD. *Handbook of Fractures, 2nd Edition.* Philadelphia: Lippincott Williams & Wilkins, 2001.)

Anatomy

- Supracondylar humerus
  - Separated into medial and lateral columns
  - Roughly triangular cross-section
  - Articular surface of the capitellum and trochlea are angled 45 degrees anteriorly
  - Neurovascular structures
    - Ulnar nerve courses subcutaneously posterior to medial epicondyle
    - Radial nerve courses posterior to lateral epicondyle
    - Brachial artery and median nerve are anterior to the elbow at the level of the antecubital fossa
- Elbow dislocations
  - Modified hinge joint
  - Normal range of motion
    - Flexion/extension: 0 to 150 degrees
    - Supination/pronation: 85 degrees/80 degrees
  - Stability
    - Anterior/posterior: Ulnohumeral bony articulation
    - Valgus: Anterior bundle of medial collateral ligament, radial head
    - Varus: Ulnohumeral bony articulation, lateral ulnar collateral ligament
- Olecranon
  - Triceps tendon inserts posteriorly
  - Subcutaneus location
  - Combines with coronoid to form the articular surface
  - Ulnar nerve exits cubital tunnel and courses immediately medial to olecranon

Model configuration

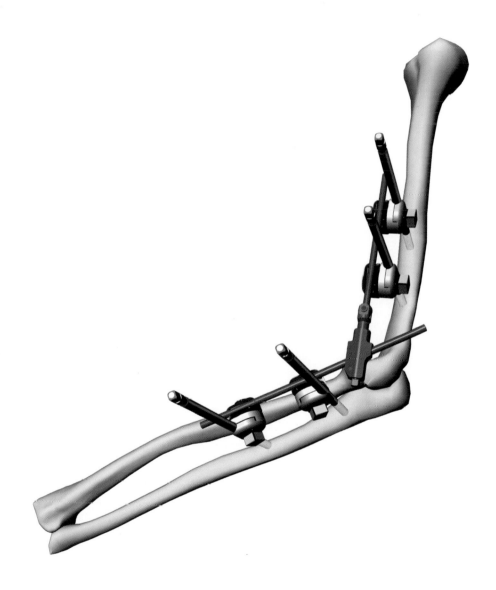

Pin placements as shown are for illustrative purposes only. Actual external fixation frame configurations and pin placements will be dependent on the clinical situation, local anatomy and the surgeon's discretion.

Safe zones and pitfalls

The purpose of elbow spanning external fixation is to provide dynamic stability by placing a pin across the distal humerus through the axis of rotation. The axis of rotation of the distal humerus runs from the bony origin of the lateral collateral ligament through the anterior/inferior aspect of the medial epicondyle.

- Distal humerus
  - Diaphyseal half-pins are placed anterolaterally
    - Care is taken to not penetrate posterior cortex where radial nerve courses in spiral groove
  - Ulnar nerve susceptible to injury if transfixion pin or axis pin is placed in lateral to medial direction through distal humeral axis of rotation
    - Avoid olecranon fossa and radial nerve

- Proximal forearm
  - Half-pins or transfixation pins are placed in a lateral to medial direction along the subcutaneus border of the ulna
  - Anterior or medial cortical violation places ulnar nerve at risk
  - Radial pins are not recommended because of risk to the posterior interosseus nerve

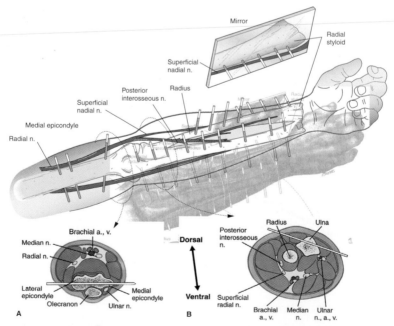

▲**Figure 6.** (Adapted from Hoppenfeld S MD. DeBoer P, MA, FRCS. *Surgical Exposures in Orthopedics: The Anatomic Approach, 3rd Edition.* Philadelphia: Lippincott Williams & Wilkins, 2003.)

External fixator construct components

DJD II body	1
4-mm half-pin	4
Pin-to-rod clamp	4

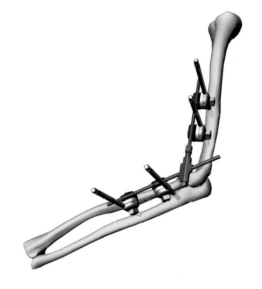

Alternative configurations

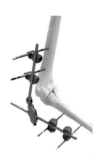

▲**Figure 7.** Unilateral (medial) Frame

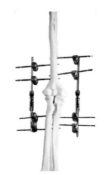

▲**Figure 8.** Bilateral Frame

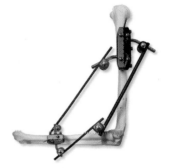

▲**Figure 9.**

Pin placements as shown are for illustrative purposes only. Actual external fixation frame configurations and pin placements will be dependent on the clinical situation, local anatomy and the surgeon's discretion.

Chapter 3:
Forearm Fractures

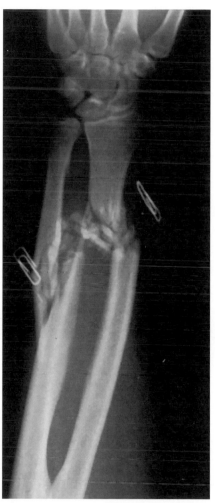
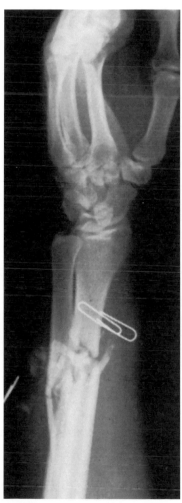

(From Chapman MW, Gordon EJ, Zissimos AG. Compression-plate fixation of acute fractures of the diaphyses of the radius and the ulna. *J Bone Joint Surg.* 1989;71A:159–169, Fig 21-27A. With permission.)

Epidemiology

- High incidence of open injuries with both bones in forearm fractures
- Increased incidence in men

Mechanism of injury

- Direct
  - Motor vehicle collision—most common
  - "Nightstick" injury
  - Gunshot wound
    - Frequently results in neurovascular injury and soft tissue deficits
- Indirect
  - Fall on outstretched hand
  - Usually from height or during athletic competition

Clinical care

- Gross deformity generally present
- Assess neurovascular status
  - Median, radial, ulnar nerves
  - Radial and ulnar arteries
- Assess soft tissue injury
- Monitor compartment pressures closely

Radiographic evaluation

- Full-length AP and lateral views of ulna and radius
- Oblique views of forearm as necessary
- Full wrist and elbow radiographs
- MRI usually not necessary
- Dynamic CT to assess DRUJ if injury suspected
- Arteriogram if arterial injury suspected

Non-operative treatment

- Nondisplaced both bones fractures are rare
  - Can be treated in a well-molded long arm cast
- Close radiographic follow-up to monitor loss of reduction

Classification system

Descriptive classification system used most commonly

- Anatomic location
  - Proximal third
  - Proximal/middle
  - Middle third
  - Middle/distal
  - Distal third
- Presence of comminution or butterfly
- Configuration
  - Transverse
  - Spiral
  - Oblique
  - Bone loss
- Angulation
  - Varus/valgus
  - Anterior/posterior
- Translation (percentage of cortical contact)
- Shortening
- Rotation
- Open versus closed

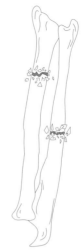

▲**Figure 2.** Transverse midshaft both bones forearm fracture

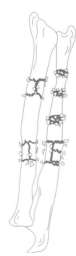

▲**Figure 3.** Comminuted both bones forearm fracture

Anatomy

- Radius and ulna form ring
  - Fracture to radius or ulna leads to fracture or dislocation of the other bone at the proximal or distal radioulnar joint
  - Examples

* Monteggia fracture: Proximal ulna fracture with radial head dislocation
* Galeazzi fracture: Distal radial shaft fracture with disruption of the DRUJ

  - "Nightstick" fractures of ulna are an exception

- "Straight" ulna acts as an axis around which the laterally bowed radius rotates in supination and pronation
- Interosseus membrane (IOM) connects the radial and ulnar diaphyses
  - Transfers loads from the distal radius to the proximal ulna
  - Fractures with associated injury to the IOM can result in instability

* Essex-Lopresti: Radial head fracture, disruption of the DRUJ, and rupture of the IOM

- Vasculature
  - Radial artery runs in the forearm on pronator teres deep to the brachioradialis
  - Ulnar artery courses proximally between FDS and FDP
- Nerves
  - Posterior interosseus nerve splits the supinator and wraps around the radial head
  - Median nerve courses medial to the brachial artery through pronator teres
  - Ulnar nerve enters between the two heads of the FCU and runs between FCU and FDP
- Surrounded by three compartments
  - Mobile wad
  - Anterior
  - Posterior

Model configuration

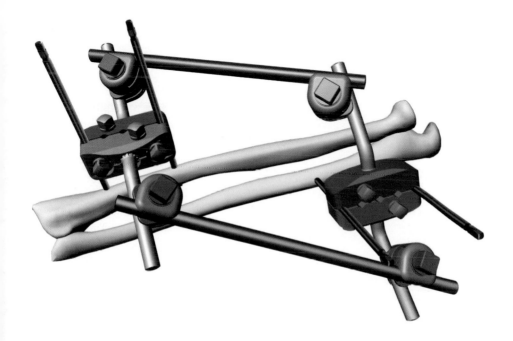

Pin placements as shown are for illustrative purposes only. Actual external fixation frame configurations and pin placements will be dependent on the clinical situation, local anatomy and the surgeon's discretion.

Safe zones and pitfalls

The relationships of the neurovascular supply relative to the radius and the ulna are fundamentally different and pin placement required for each bone is distinct. The ulna is easily palpable along its subcutaneous border. The radial artery and sensory branch of the radial nerve course through the forearm over the anterolateral aspect of the radius.

- Proximal third (see "A")
  - Ulna
    - Half-pins or transfixation pins are inserted transversely across the proximal portion
    - Ulnar nerve needs to be avoided near elbow
  - Radius
    - Pin placement not recommended because of the variable location of the posterior interosseous nerve
- Middle third (see "B")
  - Ulna
    - Half-pins or transverse pins can be placed over the subcutaneous border
  - Radius
    - Half-pins can be placed dorsally without major risk

- Distal third (see "C")
  - Ulna
    - Half-pins and transfixation pins can be placed through the subcutaneus border with minimal risk of injury to neurovascular structures
  - Radius
    - Lateral half-pins can be inserted through the distal radius posterior to the radial artery
    - Superficial radial nerve at risk
      Incision, dissection, and identification of nerve before pin placement recommended

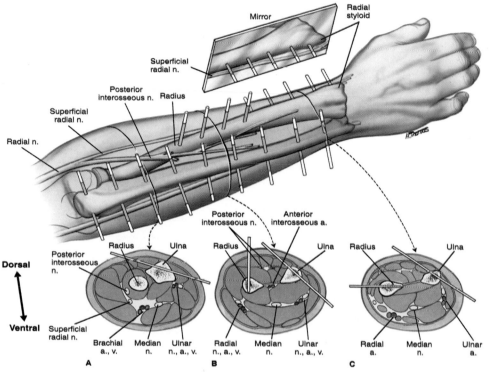

▲Figure 5. (From Hoppenfeld S, MD, DeBoer P, MA, FRCS. *Surgical Exposures in Orthopedics: The Anatomic Approach, 3rd Edition.* Philadelphia: Lippincott Williams & Wilkins, 2003.)

External fixator construct components

8-mm Connecting Rod	2
4-mm half-pin	4
Multi-pin clamp assembly	2
30-degree Angled post	4
Rod-to-rod clamp	4

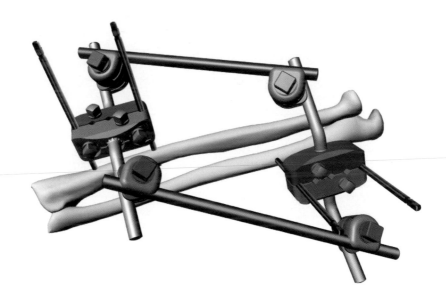

Pin placements as shown are for illustrative purposes only. Actual external fixation frame configurations and pin placements will be dependent on the clinical situation, local anatomy and the surgeon's discretion.

Alternative configurations

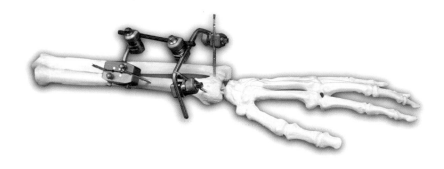

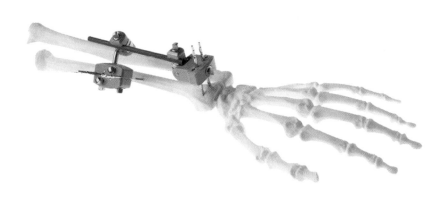

Pin placements as shown are for illustrative purposes only. Actual external fixation frame configurations and pin placements will be dependent on the clinical situation, local anatomy and the surgeon's discretion.

Chapter 4:
Wrist Fractures

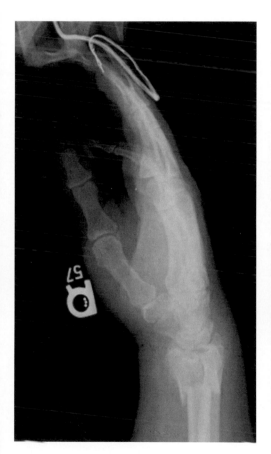

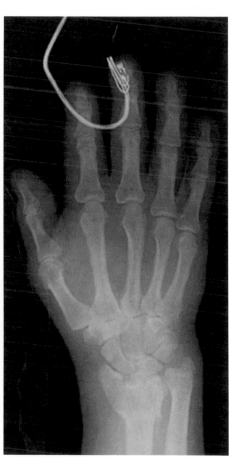

Epidemiology

- Distal radius fractures are among the most common fractures of the upper extremity
- Incidence in elderly correlates with osteoporosis

Mechanism of injury

- Low-energy (e.g., fall on outstretched hand with wrist in dorsiflexion)
  - Distal radius fails in tension over the volar aspect
  - Fracture propagates dorsally
- High-energy (e.g., motor vehicle collision)
  - Comminuted
  - Unstable

Clinical care

- Assess neurovascular status
  - Median nerve
    - Acute carpal tunnel syndrome
  - Radial and ulnar arteries
- Assess soft tissue injury

Radiographic evaluation

- AP and lateral views of the wrist
- Ipsilateral elbow radiographs
- CT can be helpful in defining intra-articular fracture pattern
- MRI usually not necessary

Nonoperative treatment

- Closed reduction and treatment with a sugar-tong splint is appropriate for stable, nondisplaced, or minimally displaced fractures meeting the following criteria:
  - Radial inclination 13 to 30 degrees (normal 22 degrees)
  - Radial height 8 to 18 millimeters (normal 11 millimeters)
  - Volar tilt 1 to 21 degrees (normal 11 degrees)
- Conversion to long arm cast for definitive treatment with frequent radiographic follow-up

Classification system

No single useful classification system. Descriptive classification system used most commonly
- Open versus closed
- Displacement
- Angulation
- Comminution
- Loss of radial height
- Intraarticular versus extraarticular

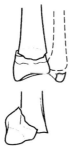

▲**Figure 2.** Extra-articular distal radius fracture with minimal shortening

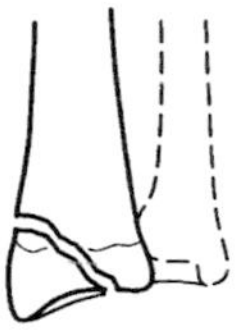

▲**Figure 3.** Intra-articular distal radius fracture

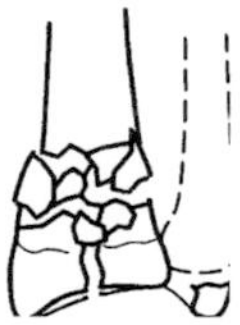

▲**Figure 4.** Complex distal intra-articular fracture with minimal displacement

Figures 2–4: (From Bucholtz RW, Heckman JD, MD. *Rockwood & Green's Fractures in Adults, 5th Edition.* Philadelphia: Lippincott Williams & Wilkins, 2002.)

Anatomy

- Metaphysis of the distal radius is predominantly cancellous bone and therefore is extremely susceptible to fracture in patients with generalized osteopenia
- 80% of the axial load is supported by the distal radius
- Range of motion
  - 160 degrees of flexion and extension
  - 180 degrees of forearm rotation
  - 50 degrees of radial and ulnar deviation
- Distal radioulnar joint (DRUJ)
  - Radial articulation with ulna at the sigmoid notch
  - Stabilized by the triangular fibrocartilage complex (TFCC)
- The radial and ulnar artery run volar to the distal radius
- The carpal canal, containing the median nerve and the flexor tendons, is volar to the distal radius
  - Median nerve at risk for acute carpal tunnel syndrome
    - Forced hyperextension
    - Fracture fragments
    - Acute hematoma

Model configuration

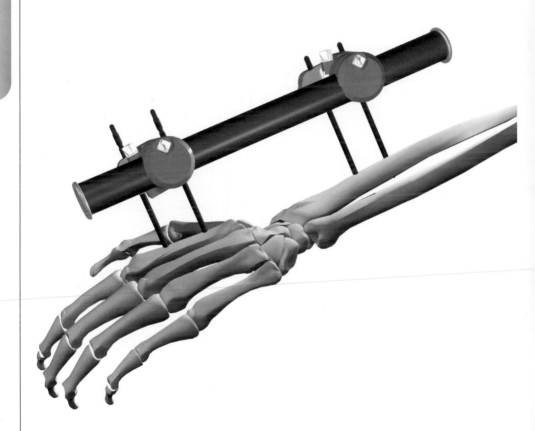

Pin placements as shown are for illustrative purposes only. Actual external fixation frame configurations and pin placements will be dependent on the clinical situation, local anatomy and the surgeon's discretion.

Safe zones and pitfalls

External fixation has grown in popularity for the treatment of distal radius fractures. Ligamentotaxis can restore radial height and inclination but rarely restores palmar tilt and does little to restore intra-articular depressed fragments. External fixation can be used to distract the fracture site, affording a better reduction, but care should be taken not to overdistract the fracture. External fixation is often supplemented with percutaneous pinning to stabilize comminuted or articular fragments.

- Distal radius
  - Lateral half-pins can be inserted through the distal radius posterior to the radial artery
  - Superficial radial nerve at risk
    - Incision, dissection, and identification of nerve before pin placement recommended
  - Interval for limited incision is between brachioradialis and FCR
- Index metacarpal
  - Distal half-pins inserted into base of index metacarpal
  - Limited dorsoradial incision at base of index metacarpal
    - Terminal branches of radial sensory nerve should be identified and retracted
    - First dorsal interosseous muscle can be sharply elevated off base of index metacarpal
      * Allows for direct access and visualization of metaphyseal flare and proximal shaft of index metacarpal

  - Half-pins are inserted at 45-degree angle to base of index metacarpal with purchase of two cortices
  - The more proximal of the distal half pins can be drilled to obtain purchase in the radial aspect the long finger metacarpal cortex
- Increased risk of overdistraction leading to difficulty with finger flexion

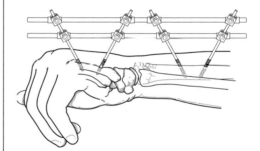

▲**Figure 6.** (From Bucholtz RW, Heckman, JD, MD. *Rockwood & Green's Fractures in Adults, 5th Edition.* Philadelphia: Lippincott Williams & Wilkins, 2002.)

Pin placements as shown are for illustrative purposes only. Actual external fixation frame configurations and pin placements will be dependent on the clinical situation, local anatomy and the surgeon's discretion.

External fixator construct components

Carbon tube (yellow)	1
Triax standard pin clamp	2
3-mm pins	4

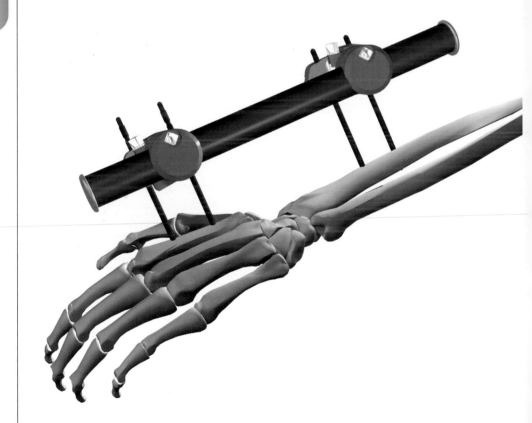

Pin placements as shown are for illustrative purposes only. Actual external fixation frame configurations and pin placements will be dependent on the clinical situation, local anatomy and the surgeon's discretion.

Alternative configurations

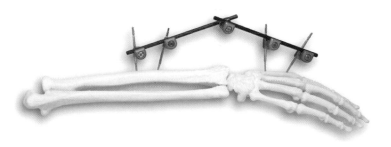

▲Figure 8.

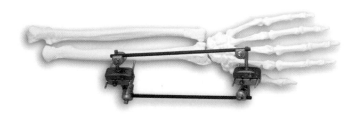

▲Figure 9.

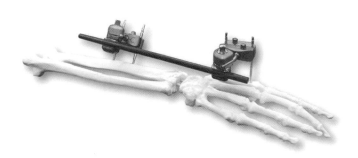

▲Figure 10.

Pin placements as shown are for illustrative purposes only. Actual external fixation frame configurations and pin placements will be dependent on the clinical situation, local anatomy and the surgeon's discretion.

Chapter 5: Hand Fractures

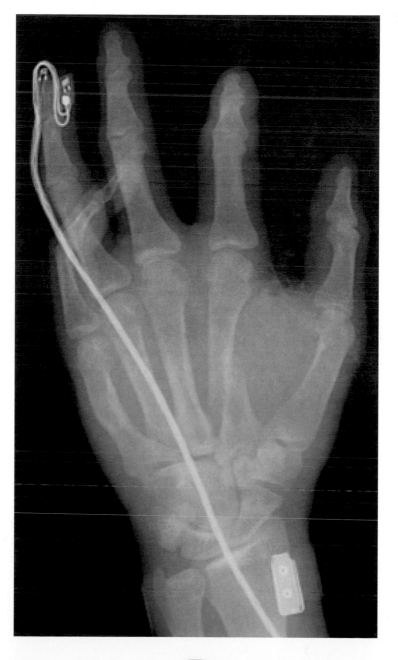

Epidemiology

- Fractures and dislocations of the metacarpal and phalanges are among the most common injuries seen in the emergency department
- Phalangeal fractures comprise 46% of all hand fractures
- Metacarpal fractures comprise 36% of all hand fractures

Mechanism of injury

- Vary considerably
- Nonepiphyseal fractures result from
  - Torque
  - Angular force
  - Compressive load
  - Direct trauma
- Epiphyseal injuries result from
  - Avulsion
  - Sheer
  - Splitting

Clinical care

- Assess neurovascular status
  - Capillary refill
  - 2-point discrimination
- Assess range of motion and rotational deformity
- Assess soft tissue injury
- Urgent reduction of dislocated joint if necessary

Radiographic evaluation

- AP, lateral, and oblique images of the affected hand or finger
- CT can be considered for intra-articular fractures
- MRI usually not necessary

Nonoperative treatment

- Reduction and immobilization is the appropriate treatment for the majority of nondisplaced extra-articular fractures or minimally, but stable, intra-articular fractures
  - Maintaining normal cascade during finger flexion is important
- Early mobilization is essential for maintaining function of affected digit

Classification system

Descriptive classification system used most commonly

- Open versus closed
- Bone involved
- Anatomic location
  - Proximal phalanx
  - Middle phalanx
  - Distal phalanx
  - Metacarpal
- Fracture pattern
  - Transverse
  - Spiral
  - Split
  - Comminuted
- Rotation
- Articular involvement
- Stability
- Dislocation
  - Determined by location of distal bone relative to proximal
    - Dorsal versus volar
    - Ulnar versus radial

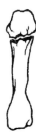

▲**Figure 2.** Oblique midshaft index metacarpal fracture

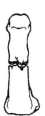

▲**Figure 4.** Transverse minimally displaced middle phalanx fracture

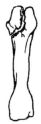

▲**Figure 3.** Intra-articular metacarpal head fracture

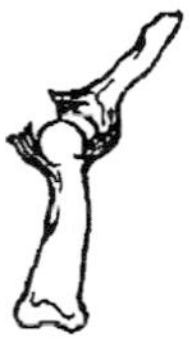

▲**Figure 5.** Dorsal distal interphalangeal phalanx dislocation with no associated fractures

Figures 2–5: (From Bucholtz RW, Heckman JD, MD. *Rockwood & Green's Fractures in Adults, 5th Edition*. Philadelphia: Lippincott Williams & Wilkins, 2002.)

Anatomy

- The metacarpophalangeal and interphalangeal joints are saddle-shaped hinge joints
- Stability is conferred by the following structures
  - Volar plate
  - Collateral ligaments
  - Joint capsule
- Neurovascular structures
  - Common digital artery runs through the palm and divides into two digital arteries
    - Travel along the radial and ulnar aspects of each digit closer to the volar surface
  - Common digital nerve follows the course of the digital artery

- Tendons
  - Flexor tendons
    - FDP and FDS course within their sheath on the volar aspect of the metacarpals and phalanges
    - Only the FDP inserts on the distal phalanx after it splits
  - Extensor tendons
    - The digital extensor tendons course through the fourth compartment of the wrist
    - Run over the dorsal aspect of each digit
    - Completes its course as the central slip
- Intrinsic muscles of the hand
  - Interossei muscles
    - Dorsal
    - Palmar
  - Lumbricals

Model configuration

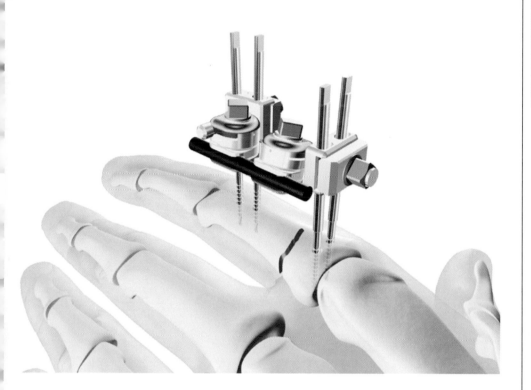

Pin placements as shown are for illustrative purposes only. Actual external fixation frame configurations and pin placements will be dependent on the clinical situation, local anatomy and the surgeon's discretion.

Safe zones and pitfalls

Oblique, spiral, and comminuted fractures of the metacarpal or phalangeal shaft are often unstable and require operative fixation. Unstable joints can also be reduced and spanned after dislocation with an external fixator.

- Metacarpals
  - Half-pins are placed dorsal to volar at a 45-degree angle to shaft axis
    - Direct dorsal placement will impair excursion of the extensor tendon
  - Limited dorsally based incision with dissection to bone allows adequate visualization for pin placement
    - Extensor tendon should be retracted
    - Common digital neurovascular bundle should be avoided

  - Bicortical purchase should be obtained without overpenetration of distal cortex
    - Potential irritation of flexor tendons or neurovascular bundle with errant placement
- Phalanges
  - Placement technique similar to metacarpals
  - Care is taken to not injure the digital neurovascular bundle along its palmar course on either side of the phalanx

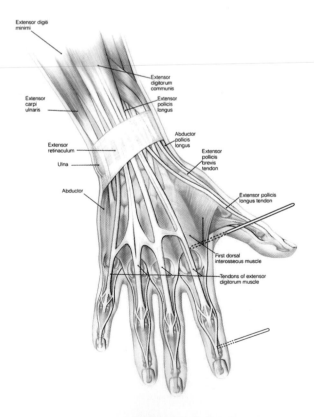

External fixator construct components

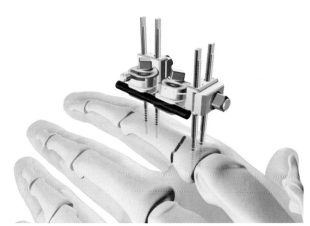

Multi-pin clamps	2
Rod-to-rod couplings	2
Connecting rod	I
2-mm half-pins	4

Alternative configurations

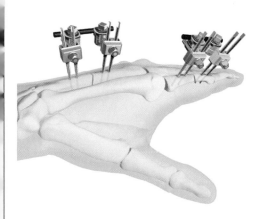

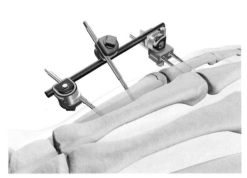

Pin placements as shown are for illustrative purposes only. Actual external fixation frame configurations and pin placements will be dependent on the clinical situation, local anatomy and the surgeon's discretion.

Chapter 6:
Pelvic Fractures

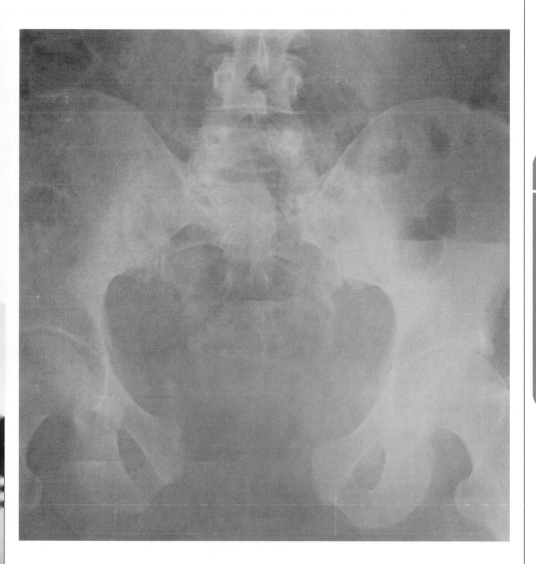

Epidemiology
- One of the few life-threatening injuries in orthopedics
- High rate of concomitant musculoskeletal and visceral injuries

Mechanism of injury
- Usually high-energy (e.g., motorcycle accidents)
  - Injury patterns vary by direction of force application
  - Lateral compression most common
    - Impaction of cancellous bone through SI joint and sacrum
    - Force applied to posterior half of the ilium results in stable configuration with minimal soft tissue injury
    - Force applied to anterior half of iliac wing results in internal rotation of hemipelvis
  - Anterior posterior force
    - External rotation of the hemipelvis hinging on posterior ligaments
  - Vertical shear
    - Vertically or longitudinally applied force (e.g., falls)
    - Complete disruption of pelvic ligaments
    - Unstable

Clinical care
- Full trauma evaluation critical
  - Airway, breathing, circulation, disability, exposure
  - Aggressive fluid resuscitation
  - Close monitoring of hemodynamic status
    - Significant blood loss should be suspected
      * Almost entire blood volume can be lost into pelvis
    - Pelvic venous plexus often disrupted
    - Less commonly, large arterial vessels may be responsible

- Immediate reduction of pelvic volume for open-book injuries
  - Emergent placement of external fixator or abdominal binder before any anticipated angiographic or operative procedure
- Vaginal and rectal examination mandatory to assess open pelvic fractures
- Assess for genitourinary and gastrointestinal injuries
- Full musculoskeletal examination to look for other orthopedic injuries
- Assess neurologic injury to lumbosacral plexus or nerve roots

Radiographic evaluation
- Initial AP view of the pelvis
- CT scan with fine (3-mm) axial cuts from lumbar spine through lesser trochanters
  - Imaging study of choice to assess posterior elements
  - 3-D reconstruction views allow for preoperative planning
- Pelvic inlet/outlet views to determine AP and superior/inferior displacement
- Iliac and obturator oblique (Judet) views to assess acetabular injuries
- MRI usually not necessary
- Arteriogram frequently required in patients who remain hemodynamically unstable after pelvic immobilization

Nonoperative treatment
- Stable minimally displaced fractures of the pelvic ring (e.g., Tile A2) can be treated conservatively with protected weight bearing
- Open-book injuries with less than 2.5 cm of pubic symphyseal diastasis can be treated with protected weight-bearing and pain control
- Lateral compression patterns resulting from forces through the posterior ilium do not require stabilization

Classification system

- Young and Burgess classification system based on mechanism of injury (Figure 2)
  - Lateral compression
  - Anterior-posterior
  - Vertical shear
- Tile classification based on direction patterns of pelvic disruption and radiographic signs of instability (Figure 3)
  - Type A: Stable
  - Type B: Rotationally unstable, vertically stable
  - Type C: Rotational and vertically unstable

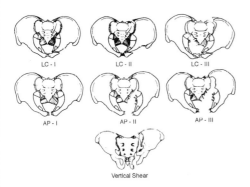

▲Figure 2. Young and Burgess classification system for pelvic fractures (From Koval KJ, MD, Zuckerman JD, MD. *Handbook of Fractures, 2nd Edition.* Philadelphia: Lippincott Williams & Wilkins, 2001.)

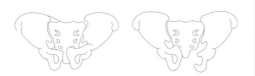

▲Figure 3. Types B and C pelvic fractures as classified by Tile (Adapted from Tile M, MD, BSc(Med), FRCS(C), Helfet DL, MD Kellam JF MD, FRCS(C). *Fractures of the Pelvis and Acetabulum, 3rd Edition.* Philadelphia: Lippincott Williams & Wilkins, 2003.)

Anatomy

- Pelvic ring is formed by the sacrum and two innominate bones
  - Joined anteriorly by the pubic symphysis
  - Joined posteriorly by the sacroiliac joints
- The innominate bone is composed of the ilium, ischium, and pubis
- Stability is maintained by ligamentous structures
  - Pubic symphysis anteriorly
  - Posterior sacroiliac ligaments
  - Sacrospinous ligaments
  - Sacrotuberous ligaments
- Bladder and genitourinary tract, as well as lower gastrointestinal tract, are contained within the pelvis
- Neurovascular structures
  - Internal and external iliac vessels are the most susceptible large vessels to pelvic injury
  - Lumbosacral plexus (T12 to S4) also at risk for damage
    - L5-S1 most commonly involved
  - Lateral femoral cutaneous nerve crosses pelvic brim within 2 cm of anterior superior iliac spine

2

PELVIS

Model configuration

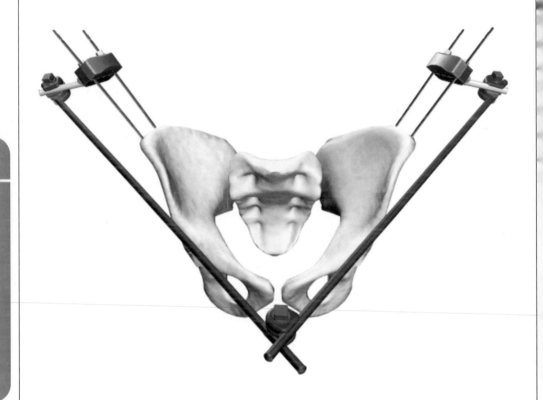

Pin placements as shown are for illustrative purposes only. Actual external fixation frame configurations and pin placements will be dependent on the clinical situation, local anatomy and the surgeon's discretion.

Safe zones and pitfalls

Pelvic external fixators are commonly used because of their rapid application in times of hemodynamic compromise and their ability to allow for access to the abdomen and pelvic viscera for secondary procedures. External fixation is most applicable to open-book pelvic fractures in which the posterior structures are intact or lateral compression injuries where there is internal rotation of the hemipelvis.

- Half-pins should be inserted into the iliac wing
  - Pins should be angled between inner and outer table
  - Violation of either cortex will decrease stability of construct
  - Penetration of medial cortex places pelvic viscera at risk

- Pins should be placed more than 2 cm posterior to anterior-superior iliac spine
  - Dissection should be carried to bone to limit risk of injury to lateral femoral cutaneous nerve

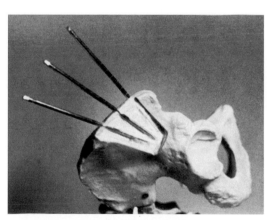

▲**Figure 5.** (Adapted from Tile M, MD, BSc(Med), FRCS(C), Helfet DL, MD Kellam JF MD, FRCS(C). *Fractures of the Pelvis and Acetabulum, 3rd Edition.* Philadelphia: Lippincott Williams & Wilkins, 2003.)

2

PELVIS

External fixator construct components

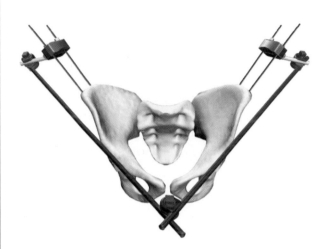

8-mm Connecting rod	2
5-mm half-pin	4
Multi-pin clamp assembly	2
30-degree Angled post	2
Rod-to-rod clamp	3

Alternative configurations

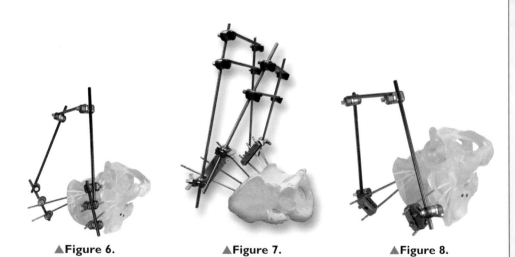

▲Figure 6. ▲Figure 7. ▲Figure 8.

Pin placements as shown are for illustrative purposes only. Actual external fixation frame configurations and pin placements will be dependent on the clinical situation, local anatomy and the surgeon's discretion.

Chapter 7:
Femoral Shaft Fractures

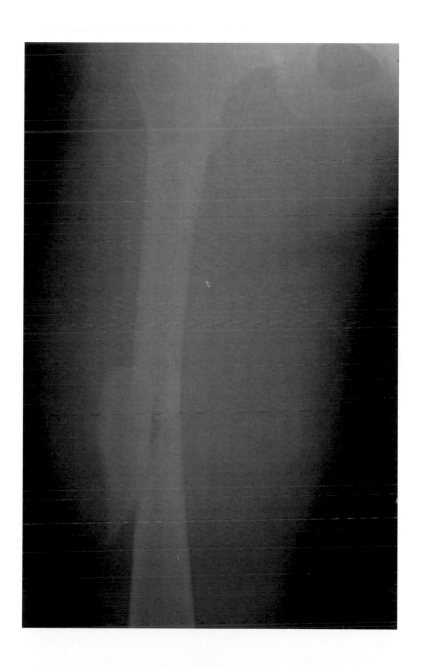

Epidemiology
- Major cause of morbidity and mortality in high-energy trauma
- 50% ligamentous and meniscal injuries in ipsilateral knee
- 5% to 15% associated injuries

Mechanism of injury
- High energy (e.g., motor vehicle collisions)
  - Most common mechanism
- Pathologic (e.g., lung cancer metastasis)
  - Elderly patients
  - Low-energy mechanism
  - Occurs at weak diaphyseal/metaphyseal junction
- Stress fracture (e.g., overuse injury in runner)
  - Often proximal to femoral midshaft region

Clinical care
- Assess neurovascular status
  - Dorsalis pedis artery
  - Posterior tibial artery
  - Sciatic and femoral nerves
- Assess soft tissue injury
- Monitor compartment pressures
- Through evaluation of involved extremity including hip and pelvis
- Frequent hemodynamic assessment
  - Average blood loss more than 1 L because of voluminous thigh compartments
- Traction pin if delayed fixation anticipated

Radiographic evaluation
- Full-length AP and lateral views of femur
- Full knee, pelvis, and hip radiographs
  - Concomitant ipsilateral femoral neck fracture occurs 3% of the time
- CT/MRI usually not necessary
- Arteriogram if arterial injury suspected

Nonoperative treatment
- Rarely indicated
- Traction or cast bracing of historical note before modern fixation techniques

Classification system

Descriptive classification system used most commonly

- Anatomic location
  - Proximal third
  - Middle third
  - Distal third
- Presence of comminution or butterfly
  - Winquist classification often used to describe degree of comminution
    - Type I: Minimal or no comminution
    - Type II: Cortices of both fragments at least 50% intact
    - Type III: 50% to 100% cortical comminution
    - Type IV: Circumferential segmental comminution
- Configuration
  - Transverse
  - Spiral
  - Oblique
  - Segmental

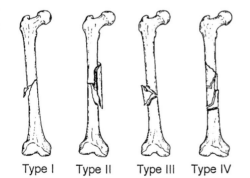

Type I   Type II   Type III   Type IV

▲**Figure 2.** Types I through IV of the Winquist classification for femur fractures (From Koval KJ, MD, Zuckerman JD, MD. *Handbook of Fractures, 2nd Edition.* Philadelphia: Lippincott Williams & Wilkins, 2001.)

- Angulation
  - Varus/valgus
  - Anterior/posterior
- Translation (percentage of cortical contact)
- Shortening
- Rotation
- Open versus closed

Anatomy

- Largest tubular bone in the body
- Anterior bow approximately 10 degrees
- Femoral shaft defined as 5 cm distal to lesser trochanter and 5 cm proximal to the adductor tubercle
- Surrounded by three compartments
  - Anterior (quadriceps, femoral vessels, and nerve)
  - Medial (adductors, obturator vessels and nerve, profunda femoris artery)
  - Posterior (hamstrings, sciatic nerve)
- Blood supply
  - Nutrient artery arising from profunda femoris artery
- Enters proximally and posteriorly along linea aspera
- Gives rise to endosteal vascular tree
  - Outer one-third of cortex supplied by periosteal vessels

Model configuration

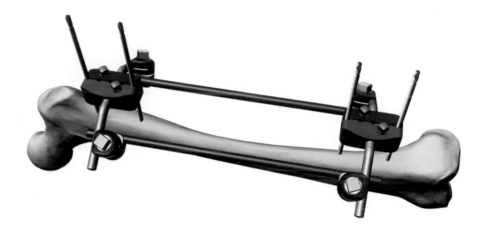

Pin placements as shown are for illustrative purposes only. Actual external fixation frame configurations and pin placements will be dependent on the clinical situation, local anatomy and the surgeon's discretion.

Safe zones and pitfalls

The femur is easily accessed with limited risk to soft tissue and neurovascular structures along its lateral border, making placement of external fixator relatively uncomplicated.

- Proximal third (see "A" below)
  - Half-pins inserted from a lateral to medial direction
  - Bicortical purchase is obtained
    - Profunda femoris artery can be injured with overpenetration of medial cortex
- Middle third (see "B" below)
  - Half-pins are usually inserted from a lateral to medial direction
  - Bicortical purchase is obtained
    - Femoral artery can be injured with overpenetration of medial cortex

- Anterior half-pins may be inserted
    - Sciatic nerve at risk with overpenetration of posterior cortex
- Distal third (see "C" below)
  - Diaphyseal half-pins are placed lateral to medial
    - Care is taken to not penetrate posterior cortex where popliteal neurovascular structures course
  - Pins should be placed proximal to condyles
    - Prevent penetration of knee joint capsule
    - Better cortical purchase

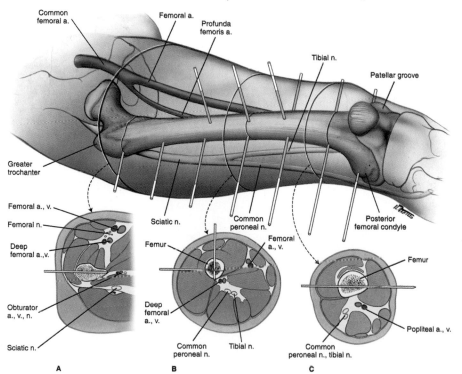

▲**Figure 4.** (From Hoppenfeld S, MD, DeBoer P, MA, FRCS. *Surgical Exposures in Orthopedics: The Anatomic Approach, 3rd Edition.* Philadelphia: Lippincott Williams & Wilkins, 2003.)

3

LOWER EXTREMITY

External fixator construct components

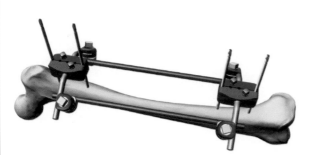

8-mm Connecting rod	2
5-mm half-pin	4
Multi-pin clamp assembly	2
30-degree Angled post	4
Rod-to-rod clamp	4

Alternative configurations

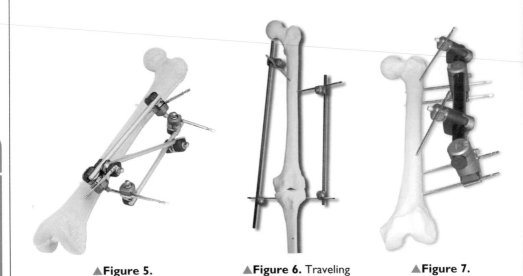

▲**Figure 5.**

▲**Figure 6.** Traveling femoral traction

▲**Figure 7.**

Pin placements as shown are for illustrative purposes only. Actual external fixation frame configurations and pin placements will be dependent on the clinical situation, local anatomy and the surgeon's discretion.

Chapter 8:
Peri-articular Knee Fractures and Dislocations

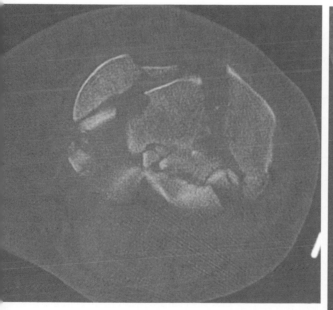

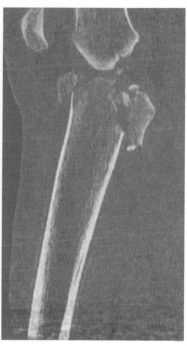

3

LOWER EXTREMITY

Epidemiology
- Distal femoral fractures
  - 7% of all femoral fractures
  - Bimodal distribution
  - Poor outcome not uncommon because of articular injury
- Knee dislocations
  - Uncommon injury
  - Limb threatening
  - Orthopedic emergency
  - Associated with muliple ligamentous injuries
- Tibial plateau fractures
  - 1% of all fractures
  - 70% to 80% are isolated to lateral plateau
  - 1% to 3% are open

Mechanism of injury
- Distal femoral fractures
  - High-energy (e.g., MVC)
    - Usually younger patients
  - Low-energy (e.g., fall on to flexed knee)
    - Most often elderly patients with osteoporotic bone
- Knee dislocations
  - High-energy (e.g., MVC)
    - Anterior dislocation produced by exaggerated hyperextension
    - Posterior dislocation usually result from posterior load to flexed knee (e.g., dashboard injury)
  - Low-energy (e.g., sports-related)
- Tibial plateau fractures
  - High-energy (e.g., MVC, bumper injury)
    - Varus or valgus stress with axial compressive force
    - Younger patients with dense bone
      * Develop split fractures
      * High rate of ligamentous injuries

- Low-energy (e.g., fall from standing)
  - Elderly with osteoporotic bone
    * Depressed or split-depressed fracture pattern
    * Low rate of ligamentous injury

Clinical care
- Full trauma evaluation
- Assess neurovascular status
  - Popliteal artery
    - 20% to 60% injury rate in knee dislocations
  - Dorsalis pedis artery
  - Posterior tibial artery
  - Peroneal nerve
    - 10% to 35% in knee dislocations
- Closed reduction if necessary
- Traction if necessary
- Assess soft tissue injury
- Monitor compartments pressures

Radiographic evaluation
- AP and lateral views of the distal femur and proximal tibia
- Radiographs of the entire affected extremity to assess concomitant injuries
- Traction x-rays often helpful in cases of intraarticular comminution
- CT essential to delineate intraarticular fracture pattern
  - Fine cuts (3 mm)
  - Sagittal and coronal reconstruction views important
  - 3-D construction useful if available
- MRI can be used to evaluate knee ligaments
- Arteriogram if arterial injury suspected
  - Low threshold for use in knee dislocations

Nonoperative treatment

- Distal femur fractures rarely treated conservatively
  - Hinged knee brace or knee immobilizer with restricted weight-bearing appropriate for the following fractures
    - Stable
    - Nondisplaced
    - Impacted
  - Skeletal traction followed by functional bracing appropriate for displaced unstable fractures in extremely poor operative candidates
- Knee dislocations
  - Emergent closed reduction
  - Reassess neurovascular status
  - Low threshold for vascular consultation
  - Range knee to assess stability
  - Immobilize at 20 to 30 degrees of flexion
  - Early ligamentous reconstruction
- Tibial plateau fractures
  - Cylinder cast or hinged knee brace suitable for closed nondisplaced fractures with articular congruity and no instability
    - Restricted weight-bearing
    - Early range of motion

Classification systems

- Distal femur fractures described by AO Müller classification (Figure 2)
  - Type A: Extraarticular
  - Type B: Unicondylar
  - Type C: Bicondylar
- Knee dislocation
  - Descriptive classification system used most commonly
    - Position of tibia relative to femur
      Anterior (most common)
      Posterior
      Medial
      Lateral
      Rotational

- Tibial Plateau fractures—Schatzker (descriptive) Classification (Figure 3)
  - Type I: Lateral plateau split
  - Type II: Lateral plateau split-depression
  - Type III: Lateral plateau depression
  - Type IV: Medial plateau
  - Type V: Bicondylar
  - Type VI: Plateau fracture with metaphyseal/diaphyseal dissociation

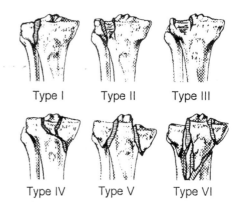

▲**Figure 3.** Tibial plateau fractures—types I through VI (From Koval KJ, MD, Zuckerman JD, MD. *Handbook of Fractures, 2nd Edition.* Philadelphia: Lippincott Williams & Wilkins, 2001.)

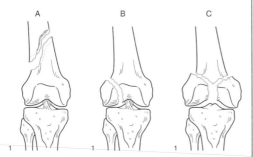

▲**Figure 2.** AO Müller types A, B, and C distal femur fractures (From Bucholtz RW, Heckman JD, MD. *Rockwood & Green's Fractures in Adults, 5th Edition.* Philadelphia: Lippincott Williams & Wilkins, 2002.)

Anatomy

- Distal femur
  - Distal 9 cm of the femur
  - Medial and lateral condyles separated by an intercondylar groove
  - Roughly trapezoidal cross section
  - Neurovascular structures
    - Popliteal artery courses posterior to the femur along with the tibial nerve
  - Fracture fragments are deformed by relative pull of quadriceps, hamstrings, and gastrocnemius
- Knee dislocations
  - Modified hinge joint
  - Three articulations
    - Patellofemoral
    - Tibiofemoral
    - Tibiofibular
  - Normal range of motion
    - Extension/flexion: -10 to 140 degrees
    - Rotation: 8 to 12 degrees
  - Stability
    - Anterior/posterior: ACL/PCL
    - Valgus/varus: MCL/LCL
    - Rupture of three out of four major ligaments necessary for dislocation
    - Multiple secondary soft tissue stabilizers of knee (e.g., menisci and capsule)
  - Vasculature
    - The five geniculate vessels branch from the popliteal artery within the popliteal fossa
    - Popliteal neurovascular bundle can be tethered during a dislocation as it courses through the fibrous tunnel at the adductor hiatus
- Tibial plateau
  - Tibia accounts for 85% of weight-bearing load
  - Medial and lateral plateau separated by intercondylar eminence
  - Medial and lateral menisci rest on the articular surface
  - Three bony prominences exist within 3 cm distal to the plateau
    - Tibial tubercle: Anterior insertion of patellar tendon
    - Pes anserinus: Medial attachment for hamstrings
    - Gerdy's tubercle: Lateral attachment of iliotibial band
  - Knee capsule extends 14 mm distal to articular surface
  - Peroneal nerve exits popliteal fossa and courses subcutaneously around fibular head

3

Model configuration

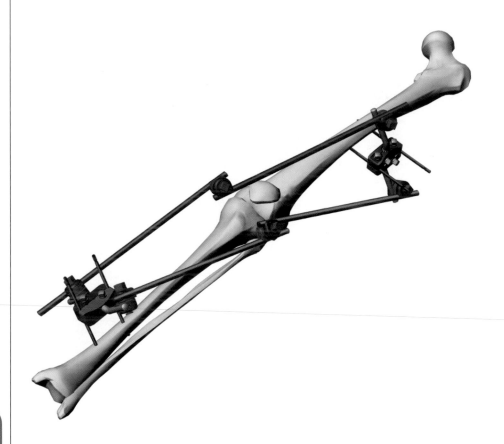

Pin placements as shown are for illustrative purposes only. Actual external fixation frame configurations and pin placements will be dependent on the clinical situation, local anatomy and the surgeon's discretion.

Safe zones and pitfalls

Thin cortices, frequent comminution, wide medullary canal, and osteopenia make internal fixation difficult in the distal femur and the proximal tibia. Joint spanning external fixation is often useful when rapid stabilization of fractures is necessary because of soft tissue concerns or vascular compromise. For patients with significant comminution, a hybrid ring external fixator may be placed. The advantages to a ring fixator include multiplanar adjustments and increased stability in articular comminution. However, complexity in application and obstruction of soft tissue may limit its use.

- Distal femur
  - Diaphyseal half-pins are placed lateral to medial
    - Care is taken to not penetrate posterior cortex where popliteal neurovascular structures course
  - Pins should be placed proximal to condyles
    - Prevent penetration of knee joint capsule
    - Better cortical purchase

- Proximal tibia
  - Anterior tibial artery located anterior to interosseous membrane
  - Posterior tibial artery lies behind the tibialis posterior muscle
  - Half-pins should be inserted anterior to posterior through the subcutaneus surface of the bone
  - Transfibular transfixion pins cannot be inserted at this level
  - Posteriorly directed transfixion pins are to be avoided
  - Pins should be placed more than 14 mm distal from the tibial articular surface to avoid penetration of the joint

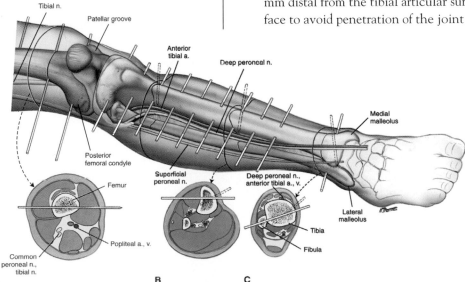

3

LOWER EXTREMITY

(Adapted from Hoppenfeld S, MD, DeBoer P, MA, FRCS. *Surgical Exposures in Orthopedics: The Anatomic Approach, 3rd Edition*. Philadelphia: Lippincott Williams & Wilkins, 2003.)

External fixator construct components

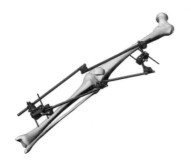

30-degree Posts	4
5-mm half-pin	4
Pin clamp assemblies	2
Rod-to-rod coupling	6
8-mm Connecting rods	4

Alternative configurations

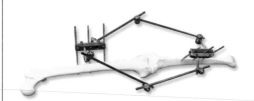

▲**Figure 6.**   ▲**Figure 7.**

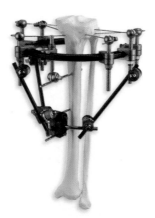

▲**Figure 8.** Hybrid external fixation

Pin placements as shown are for illustrative purposes only. Actual external fixation frame configurations and pin placements will be dependent on the clinical situation, local anatomy and the surgeon's discretion.

Chapter 9:
Tibial Shaft Fractures

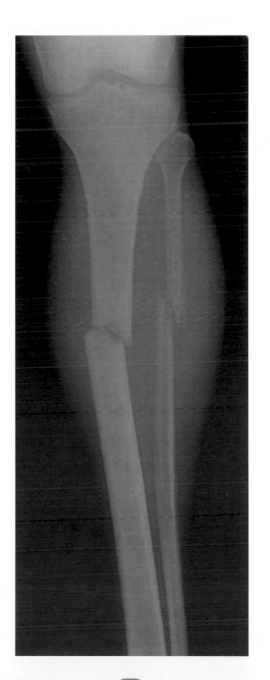

Epidemiology

- Tibial shaft most common long bone fracture
- 500,000 cases/year

Mechanism of injury

- High-energy (e.g., motor vehicle collisions)
  - Transverse
  - Comminuted
  - Displaced
  - Significant soft tissue injury
- Penetrating (e.g., gunshot wound)
  - Variable fracture pattern
  - High Velocity vs low velocity
- Bending (e.g., ski boot injuries)
  - Short, oblique
  - Transverse
  - Possible butterfly fragments
- Torsion (e.g., twisting with foot fixed)
  - Spiral, nondisplaced
  - Minimal soft tissue disruption

Clinical care

- Assess neurovascular status
  - Dorsalis pedis artery
  - Posterior tibial artery
  - Common peroneal nerve
- Assess soft tissue injury
- Monitor compartment pressures

Radiographic evaluation

- Full-length AP and lateral views of tibia
- Full knee and ankle radiographs
- CT/MRI usually not necessary
- Arteriogram if arterial injury suspected

Nonoperative treatment

- Long leg cast considered for isolated, closed low-energy fractures meeting the following criteria
  - Less than 5-degree varus/valgus angulation
  - Less than 10-degree anterior/posterior angulation
  - Less than 10-degree rotation
  - 50% cortical contact
  - Less than 1 cm of shortening
- Average time to union is 16 ± 4 weeks

Classification system

Descriptive classification system used most commonly

- Anatomic location
  - Proximal third
  - Middle third
  - Distal third
- Presence of comminution or butterfly
- Configuration
  - Transverse
  - Spiral
  - Oblique
  - Segmental
- Angulation
  - Varus/valgus
  - Anterior/posterior
- Translation (percentage of cortical contact)
- Shortening
- Rotation
- Open versus closed
  - Gustilo classification used for open injuries

Gustilo classification system for open fractures

- Type I
  - Clean wound
  - Less than 1 cm in length
- Type II
  - Wound between 1 and 10 cm in length
  - Limited soft tissue damage
- Type III
  - Wounds larger than 10 cm
  - Extensive soft tissue damage
  - IIIA
    - Adequate soft tissue to cover bone
  - IIIB
    - Exposed bone requiring extensive soft tissue repair (e.g., flap)
  - IIIC
    - Associated vascular injury requiring repair

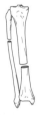

▲**Figure 2.** Minimally displaced distal third transverse tibial shaft fracture

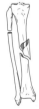

▲**Figure 4.** Middle third spiral tibial shaft fracture with medially displaced butterfly fragment

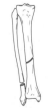

▲**Figure 3.** Minimally displaced middle third short oblique tibial shaft fracture

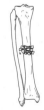

▲**Figure 5.** Comminuted mid-shaft tibia fracture with minimal displacement

Figures 2–5: (From Bucholtz RW, Heckman JD, MD. *Rockwood & Green's Fractures in Adults, 5th Edition.* Philadelphia: Lippincott Williams & Wilkins, 2002.)

3

LOWER EXTREMITY

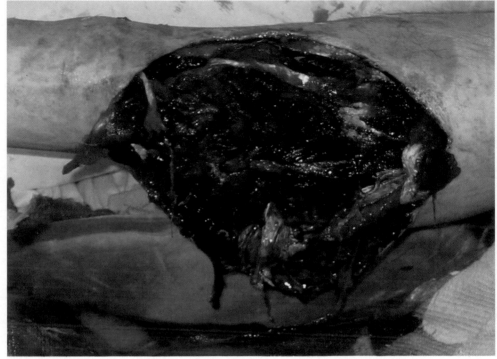

▲Figure 6. Type IIIB open tibia fracture

Anatomy

- Long tubular bone with triangular cross-sections
- Subcutaneous anteromedial border
- Surrounded by four compartments
  - Anterior (EHL, Tib ant, Per tertius, Ant tib artery, deep peroneal nerve)
  - Lateral (peroneus longus and brevis, superficial peroneal nerve)
  - Deep posterior (FHL, FDL, Tib post, posterior tibial artery and nerve)
  - Superficial posterior (Gastroc/soleus, plantaris)
- Blood supply
  - Nutrient artery arising from posterior tibial artery
    - Enters posterolateral cortex distal to soleus origin
    - Gives rise to endosteal vascular tree
  - Anterior tibial artery
  - Peroneal artery
  - Distal third supplied by periosteal anastomoses
    - Area at higher risk for nonunion
- Tibia responsible for 85% of weight-bearing load
- Common peroneal nerve at risk as it wraps subcutaneously around fibular head

Model configuration

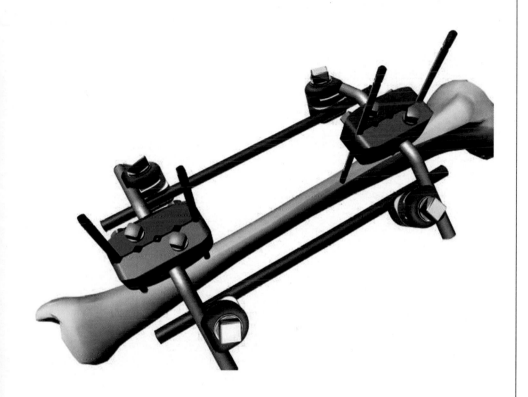

Pin placements as shown are for illustrative purposes only. Actual external fixation frame configurations and pin placements will be dependent on the clinical situation, local anatomy and the surgeon's discretion.

Safe zones and pitfalls

Because of the triangular cross-section of the tibia and the posteriorly placed neurovascular bundle, pin placement is fairly straightforward. The subcutaneous anteromedial surface of the bone can be used throughout its entire length for placement of half-pins.

- Proximal third
  - Anterior tibial artery located anterior to interosseous membrane
  - Posterior tibial artery lies behind the tibialis posterior
  - Transfibular transfixation pins cannot be inserted at this level
  - Posteriorly directed transfixion pins are to be avoided
  - Half-pins are inserted at the oblique medial aspect of tibia
- Middle third
  - Anterior tibial vessels hug the medial tibial cortex
  - Posterior neurovascular bundle continues to course betweenB in the deep compartment superficial to the tibialis posterior
  - Anterior half pins are inserted at the subcutaneous border of the tibia
- Distal third
  - Anterior tibial vessels and deep peroneal nerve
    - Cross the lateral tibial cortex
    - Wrap anteriorly becoming more vulnerable
  - Before insertion of anterior half-pins near ankle, perform blunt dissection to bone to ensure safety of neurovascular bundle

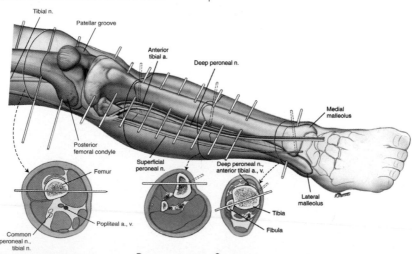

(Adapted from Hoppenfeld S, MD, DeBoer P, MA, FRCS. *Surgical Exposures in Orthopedics: The Anatomic Approach, 3rd Edition.* Philadelphia: Lippincott Williams & Wilkins, 2003.)

External fixator construct components

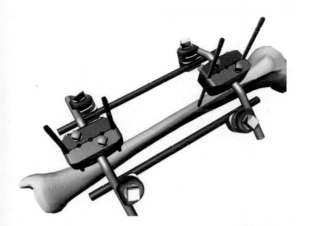

8-mm Connecting rod	2
5-mm half-pin	4
Multi-pin clamp assembly	2
30-degree Angled post	4
Rod-to-rod clamp	4

Pin placements as shown are for illustrative purposes only. Actual external fixation frame configurations and pin placements will be dependent on the clinical situation, local anatomy and the surgeon's discretion.

3

LOWER EXTREMITY

Alternative configurations

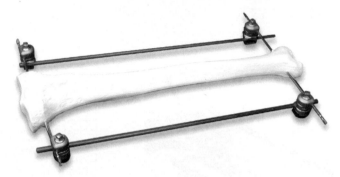

▲**Figure 10.** Traveling tibial traction

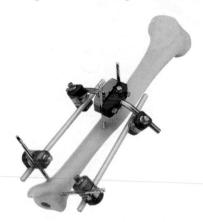

▲**Figure 11.** Distal tibia shaft fracture

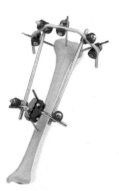

▲**Figure 12.** Semicircular frame for proximal tibia

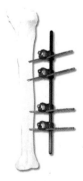

▲**Figure 13.** Independent pin for mid-shaft fracture

Pin placements as shown are for illustrative purposes only. Actual external fixation frame configurations and pin placements will be dependent on the clinical situation, local anatomy and the surgeon's discretion.

Chapter 10:
Peri-articular Ankle Fractures and Dislocations

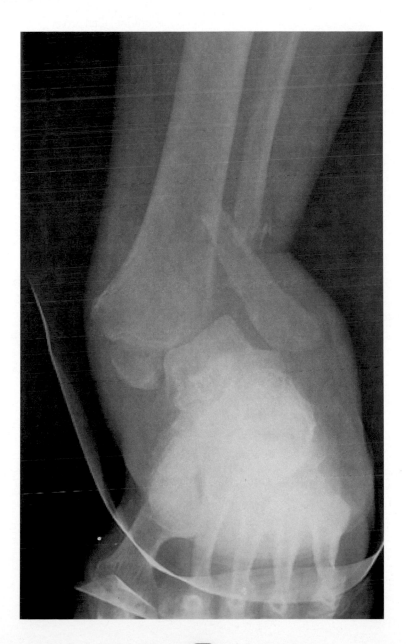

Epidemiology
- Tibial pilon (plafond) fractures
  - 7% to 10% of all tibia fractures
  - Usually significant soft tissue compromise
- Bimalleolar ankle fractures
  - Common orthopedic injury
  - Athletes at higher risk
- Subtalar dislocations
  - Infrequent
  - Significant soft tissue injury
  - Medial or lateral
  - May be associated with fractures of the talus

Mechanism of injury
- Tibial pilon fracture
  - Axial compression (e.g., fall from height)
    - Axially directed force through the talus into the plafond
    - Impaction of articular surface
  - Shear (e.g., skiing injury)
    - Torsion combined with varus or valgus stress
    - Two or more large fragments produced
    - Associated fibula fracture
- Bimalleolar fractures
  - Usually rotational injuries with specific pattern dictated by position of the foot at time of injury and direction of deforming force
- Subtalar dislocations
  - Inversion
    - Medial dislocation
  - Eversion
    - Lateral dislocation

Clinical care
- Full trauma evaluation
  - Especially with pilon fractures
    - Spine evaluation critical because of transfer of loads through axial skeleton
- Assess neurovascular status
  - Dorsalis pedis
  - Posterior tibial artery
  - Peroneal nerves
  - Posterior tibial nerve
- Closed reduction if necessary
  - Medial subtalar dislocation often blocked by capsule
  - Lateral subtalar dislocation often blocked by posterior tibial tendon
- Assess soft tissue injury
  - Tenuous soft tissue envelope can result in conversion of a closed fracture to an open fracture
  - Elevation, ice, and splinting of affected extremity essential

Radiographic evaluation
- Full-length AP, lateral, and mortise views of the ankle
- Postreduction x-rays help identify occult fractures
  - Calcaneus
  - Talus
- CT essential for pilon fractures to delineate intraarticular fracture pattern
- MRI can be used to evaluate ankle ligaments in isolated dislocations
- Arteriogram if arterial injury suspected

Nonoperative treatment

- Pilon fractures
  - Long leg cast followed by fracture brace for nondisplaced fractures with nontraumatized soft tissue envelope
  - Loss of reduction common and unable to monitor soft tissue status
  - Reserved for severely debilitated patients
- Bimalleolar fractures
  - Closed reduction for displaced fractures
  - Posterior splint with "U" component appropriate for nondisplaced stable fractures
  - Conversion to long leg cast for 4 to 6 weeks with restricted weight-bearing
- Isolated subtalar dislocations
  - Immediate closed reduction
  - Short period (4 weeks) of immobilization
  - Increase in progressive weight-bearing and range of motion exercises

Classification systems

- Pilon fracture classification as described by Ruedi-Allgöwer based on comminution and articular displacement (Figure 2)
  - Type I: Nondisplaced articular surface and nondisplaced bony fragments
  - Type II: Significant articular incongruity with minimal comminution
  - Type III: Significant articular comminution with metaphyseal impaction
- Bimalleolar fractures classified by mechanism as described by Lauge-Hansen (Figure 3)

- System first describes position of the foot at time of injury, followed by the direction of the deforming force
  - Supination—adduction
  - Supination—external rotation
  - Pronation—external rotation
  - Pronation—adduction
  - Subtalar dislocations
  - Based on position of foot relative to talus
  - Medial
  - Lateral

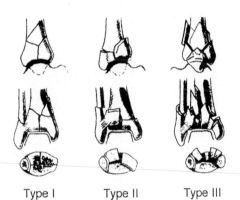

Type I   Type II   Type III

▲**Figure 2.** Ruedi-Allgöwer types I, II, and III tibial plafond fractures (From Koval KJ, MD, Zuckerman JD, MD. *Handbook of Fractures, 2nd Edition.* Philadelphia: Lippincott Williams & Wilkins, 2001.)

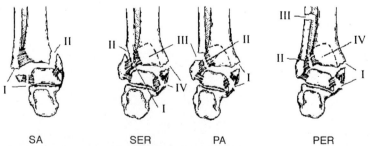

SA   SER   PA   PER

▲**Figure 3.** Lauge-Hansen ankle fracture classification system (Adapted from Koval KJ, MD, Zuckerman JD, MD. *Handbook of Fractures, 2nd Edition.* Philadelphia: Lippincott Williams & Wilkins, 2001.)

Anatomy

- Distal tibia
  - Flares out to form the plafond
  - Cortical diaphyseal bone changes to cancellous bone over articular surface
  - Articular surface wider anteriorly than posteriorly
    - Accommodates the wedge-shaped talus
  - Thin soft tissue envelope and precarious microcirculation surround the distal tibia
  - Neurovascular structures
    - Dorsalis pedis artery and deep peroneal nerve course anteriorly
    - Posterior tibial artery and tibial nerve run posteromedially through tarsal tunnel
    - Superficial peroneal nerve courses anterolaterally
- Ankle joint
  - Complex hinge joint
    - Tibiofibular
    - Tibiotalar
    - Talofibular
  - Mortise consists of the tibial plafond and both malleoli to form constrained articulation with talar dome
  - Ligaments
    - Deltoid ligament provides medial stabilization
    - Lateral ligaments (anterior and posterior talofibular and calcaneofibular) provide lateral stabilization
    - Syndesmosis ligament complex (anterior and posterior tibiofibular, interosseous ligament, transverse tibiofibular) between the tibia and fibula resists axial, translational, and rotational forces
  - Range of motion
    - Dorsiflexion: 30 degrees
    - Plantarflexion: 35 degrees
- Subtalar joint
  - Articulation between calcaneus and talar body
  - Responsible for inversion and eversion

3

Model configuration

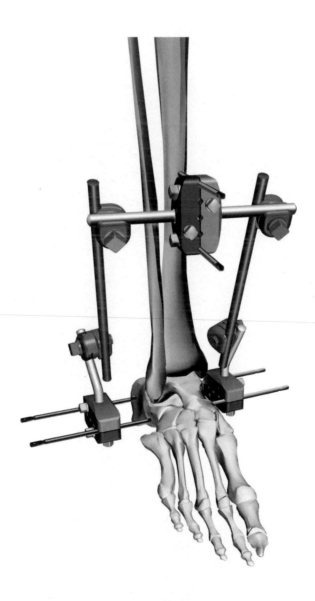

Pin placements as shown are for illustrative purposes only. Actual external fixation frame configurations and pin placements will be dependent on the clinical situation, local anatomy and the surgeon's discretion.

Safe zones and pitfalls

Joint spanning external fixation is often useful when rapid stabilization of fractures is necessary because of soft tissue concerns or vascular compromise. For isolated subtalar dislocation, external fixators are often used primarily for stabilization. For patients with significant comminution, a hybrid ring external fixator may be placed. The advantages to a ring fixator include multiplanar adjustments and increased stability in articular comminution. However, complexity in application and obstruction of soft tissue may limit its use.

- Distal third
  - Anterior tibial vessels and deep peroneal nerve
    - Cross the lateral tibial cortex
    - Wrap anteriorly becoming more vulnerable
  - Before insertion of anterior half-pins near ankle, perform blunt dissection to bone to ensure safety of neurovascular bundle

- Calcaneus
  - Transfixion pins are placed through the calcaneus from medial to lateral
    - Tibial nerve and the posterior tibial vessels course posterior to the medial malleolus through the tarsal tunnels
    - Pins are inserted distal and posterior to the bundle
      * 2 cm anterior to the posterior border of the calcaneus
      * 2 cm superior to the plantar aspect of the calcaneus

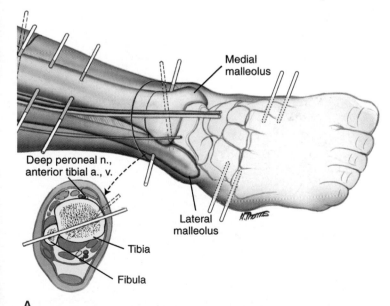

Medial malleolus

Deep peroneal n., anterior tibial a., v.

Lateral malleolus

Tibia

Fibula

A

(Adapted from Hoppenfeld S, MD, DeBoer P, MA, FRCS. *Surgical Exposures in Orthopedics: The Anatomic Approach, 3rd Edition.* Philadelphia: Lippincott Williams & Wilkins, 2003.)

3

LOWER EXTREMITY

External fixator construct components

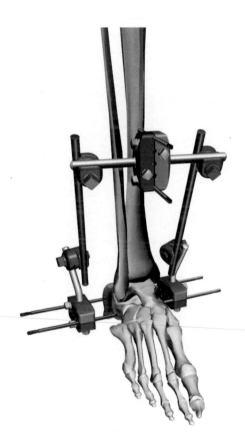

8-mm Connecting rods	2
Multi-pin clamp assembly	3
30-degree Angled posts	4
Rod-to-rod clamps	4
4-mm transfixing pins	2
5-mm half-pins	2

Pin placements as shown are for illustrative purposes only. Actual external fixation frame configurations and pin placements will be dependent on the clinical situation, local anatomy and the surgeon's discretion.

Alternative configurations

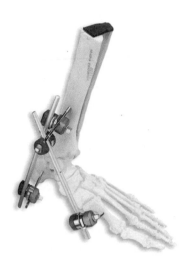

▲**Figure 6.**

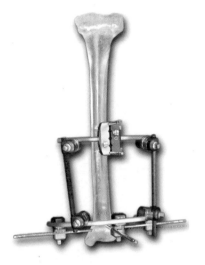

▲**Figure 7.**

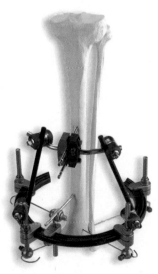

▲**Figure 8.** Hybrid external fixation

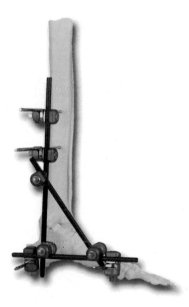

▲**Figure 9.**

Pin placements as shown are for illustrative purposes only. Actual external fixation frame configurations and pin placements will be dependent on the clinical situation, local anatomy and the surgeon's discretion.

3

LOWER EXTREMITY

Chapter 11:
Forefoot Fractures and Dislocations

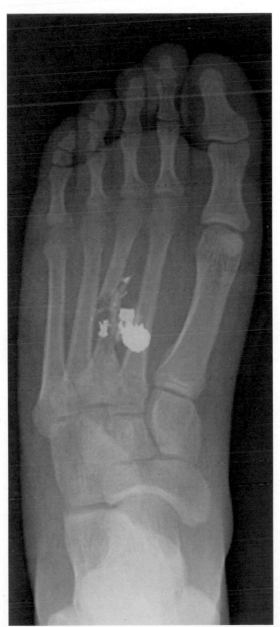

Epidemiology

- True number of metatarsal and phalangeal fractures unknown
  - Number of treating physicians (e.g., family practitioners, podiatrists, orthopedic surgeons)
- Most phalangeal fractures occur as a result of improper footwear

Mechanism of injury

- Vary considerably
- Nonepiphyseal fractures result from
  - Torque (e.g., body rotation against fixed foot)
  - Angular force
  - Axial load (e.g., stubbing)
  - Direct trauma (e.g., dropped objects)
  - Stress fractures
- Epiphyseal injuries result from
  - Avulsion
  - Sheer
  - Splitting

Clinical care

- Assess neurovascular status
- Assess rotational deformity
- Assess soft tissue injury
- Assess weight-bearing capacity and mobility
- Rule out Lisfranc dislocation of midfoot
- Urgent reduction of dislocated joint if necessary

Radiographic evaluation

- AP, lateral, and oblique images of the affected foot or toe
- Stress views of foot for suspected Lisfranc injuries
- Bone scan for occult fractures
- MRI for infection or ligamentous injuries

Nonoperative treatment

- Reduction and immobilization is the appropriate treatment for the majority of nondisplaced extraarticular fractures or minimally, but stable, intra-articular fractures
  - Short-leg walking cast or nonweight-bearing cast for 2 to 4 weeks for metatarsal fractures
  - Buddy taping and rigid sole orthosis for phalangeal injuries and dislocations

Classification system

Descriptive classification system used most commonly

- Open versus closed
- Bone involved
- Anatomic location
  - Proximal phalanx
  - Middle phalanx
  - Distal phalanx
  - Metatarsal
- Fracture pattern
  - Transverse
  - Spiral
  - Split
  - Comminuted
- Rotation
- Articular involvement
- Stability
- Dislocation
  - Determined by location of distal bone relative to proximal
    - Plantar versus dorsal
    - Medial versus lateral

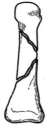

▲**Figure 2.** Spiral extra-articular metatarsal fracture

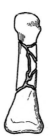

▲**Figure 3.** Comminuted extra-articular metatarsal fracture

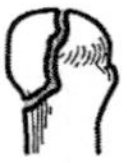

▲**Figure 4.** Intra-articular metatarsal head fracture

Figures 2–4: (From Koval KJ, MD, Zuckerman JD, MD. *Handbook of Fractures, 2nd Edition.* Philadelphia: Lippincott Williams & Wilkins, 2001.)

3

LOWER EXTREMITY

Anatomy

- The first metatarsal is larger and stronger than the lesser metatarsals
  - Shares a greater proportion of the load
  - Requires strict anatomic reduction
- The metatarsophalangeal and interphalangeal joints are saddle-shaped hinge joints
- Stability is conferred by the following structures
  - Plantar plate
  - Collateral ligaments
  - Joint capsule
- Neurovascular structures
  - Metatarsals and phalanges are supplied by an anastomosis of vessels
    - Dorsal: Dorsalis pedis artery
    - Plantar: Medial and lateral plantar arteries
  - Sensation of the dorsal aspect of the foot is supplied by the superficial peroneal nerve
    - The first webspace is supplied by the deep peroneal nerve
  - Most of the plantar sensation arises from the medial and lateral plantar nerves branching from the tibial nerve
- Tendons
  - Flexor tendons
    - FHL and FDL course on the plantar aspect of the metatarsals and phalanges
  - Extensor tendons
    - EHL and EDL run over the dorsal aspect of the ankle and foot

Model configuration

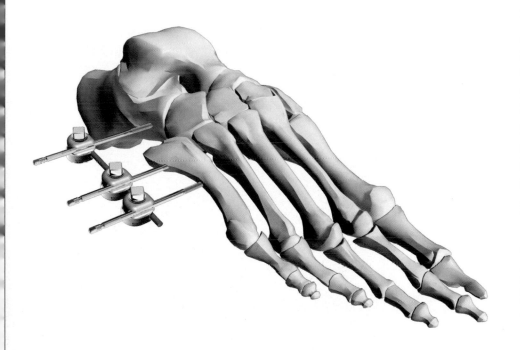

Pin placements as shown are for illustrative purposes only. Actual external fixation frame configurations and pin placements will be dependent on the clinical situation, local anatomy and the surgeon's discretion.

3

LOWER EXTREMITY

Safe zones and pitfalls

Oblique, spiral, and comminuted fractures of the metatarsal or phalangeal shaft are often unstable and require operative fixation, especially fracture of the first metatarsal. Unstable joints can also be reduced and spanned after dislocation with an external fixator.

- Metatarsals
  - Half-pins are placed dorsal to plantar at a 45-degree angle
    - Direct dorsal placement will impair excursion of the extensor tendon
  - Limited dorsally based incision with dissection to bone allows adequate visualization for pin placement
    - Extensor tendon should be retracted
    - Digital neurovascular bundle should be avoided
  - Bicortical purchase should be obtained without overpenetration of distal cortex
    - Potential irritation of flexor tendons or neurovascular bundle with errant placement
- Phalanges
  - Placement technique similar to metacarpals
  - Care is taken to not injure the digital neurovascular bundle along its plantar or dorsal course on either side of the phalanx

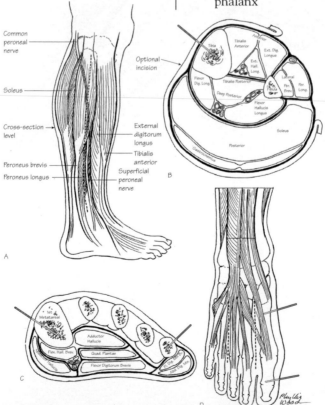

(Adapted from Hansen ST, MD. *Functional Reconstruction of the Foot and Ankle.* Philadelphia: Lippincott Williams & Wilkins. 2000.)

External fixator construct components

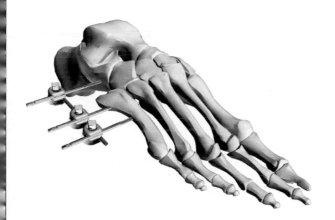

Pin-to-rod clamps	3
Connecting rod	1
3-mm half-pin	3

Alternative configurations

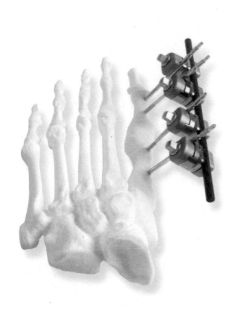

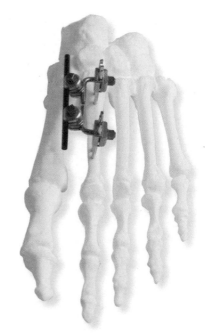

Pin placements as shown are for illustrative purposes only. Actual external fixation frame configurations and pin placements will be dependent on the clinical situation, local anatomy and the surgeon's discretion.

3

LOWER EXTREMITY

Glossary

Self Drilling/Self Tapping Half Pin: 1.65mm–6mm	
Blunt Half Pin: 2mm–6mm	
Transfixing pin: 4mm–5mm	
DJD II Body	
Multi-Pin Clamp Assemblies Large, Small & Micro sizes	
Peri-Articular Clamp	
Pin Clamp Assemblies (unilateral fixators) Large, Medium & Small sizes	
Pin-to-Rod Clamps Large, Small & Micro size	
Rod-to-Rod Clamps Large, Small & Micro sizes	
Posts	
Connecting Rods Large, Small & Micro sizes	
Carbon Rings	
Hybrid Pin Post	
Hybrid Ring Clamp	
Hybrid Wire Post	

References

Browner B, Trafton P, Green N, Swiontkowski M, Jupiter J, LevineA, eds. *Skeletal Trauma*. 3rd ed. Philadelphia, PA: Saunders, 2003.

Bucholz RW, Heckman JD, eds. *Rockwood and Green's Fractures in Adults*. 5th ed. Baltimore, MD: Lippincott Williams & Wilkins, 2002.

Canale ST, ed. *Campbell's Operative Orthopaedics*. 10th ed. New York, NY: Mosby, 2003.

Chapman MW, Szabo RM, Marder RA, Vince KG, Mann RA, Lane JM, McLain RF, Rab G, eds. *Chapman's Orthopaedic Surgery*. 3rd ed. Baltimore, MD: Lippincott Williams & Wilkins, 2000.

Craig EV, ed. *Clinical Orthopaedics*. 1st ed. Baltimore, MD: Lippincott Williams & Wilkins, 1999.

Green D, Hotchkiss R, Pederson W, eds. *Green's Operative Hand Surgery*. 4th ed. Philadelphia, PA: Churchill Livingstone, 1999.

Hansen ST, ed. *Functional Reconstruction of the Foot and Ankle*. Philadelphia, PA: Lippincott Williams & Wilkins, 2000.

Koval KJ, Zuckerman JD, eds. *Handbook of Fractures*. 2nd ed. Baltimore, MD: Lippincott Williams & Wilkins, 2001.

Rüedi T, Murph W, eds. *AO Principles of Fracture Management*. 2nd ed. New York, NY: Springer-Verlag, 2001.

Tile M, Helfet DL, Kellam JK, eds. *Fractures of the Pelvis and Acetabulum*. 3rd ed. Baltimore, MD: Lippincott Williams & Wilkins, 2003.

Wiss DA, ed. *Masters Techniques in Orthopaedic Surgery: Fractures*. 1st ed. Baltimore, MD: Lippincott Williams & Wilkins, 1998.